BREAKING THE CHAIN

BREAKING THE CHAIN

Drugs and Cycling: The True Story

WILLY VOET
TRANSLATED BY
WILLIAM FOTHERINGHAM

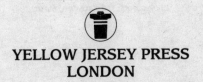

YELLOW JERSEY PRESS
LONDON

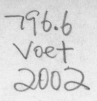

First published by Yellow Jersey Press 2001
This edition 2002

6 8 10 9 7 5

Copyright © Calmann-Lévy, 1999

Willy Voet has asserted his right under the Copyright, Designs and Patents Act
1988 to be identified as the author of this work

First published in Great Britain in 2001 by
Yellow Jersey Press
Random House, 20 Vauxhall Bridge Road,
London SW1V 2SA

Random House Australia (Pty) Limited
20 Alfred Street, Milsons Point, Sydney,
New South Wales 2061, Australia

Random House New Zealand Limited
18 Poland Road, Glenfield,
Auckland 10, New Zealand

Random House South Africa (Pty) Limited
Isle of Houghton, Corner of Boundary Road & Carse O'Gowrie,
Houghton 2198, South Africa

Random House UK Limited Reg. No. 954009

A CIP catalogue record for this book is available from the British Library

ISBN 0 224 06117 8

Papers used by Random House are natural, recyclable products made
from wood grown in sustainable forests. The manufacturing processes conform
to the environmental regulations of the country of origin

Printed and bound in Great Britain by
Bookmarque Ltd, Croydon, Surrey

For Bruno, Eric and Nathalie

CONTENTS

CONTENTS

TRANSLATOR'S NOTE

Many observers who watched the Tour de France come to the brink of collapse in July 1998 felt that in future cycling might come to be seen in two eras: before and after the Festina drugs scandal. This is borne out by events since that early morning when a French customs officer put out his arm to wave Willy Voet and his cargo of erythroporetin, growth hormone, testosterone, amphetamines and 'Belgian mix' to the side of the road, so sparking off the saga.

Since then, cycling has come under judicial scrutiny of an intensity which no other sport has ever witnessed, and the succession of investigations, trials, sentences and bans has meant that the results of an entire generation – cycling's EPO generation – have to be seen in a new light. Unfortunately, yet inevitably, it means that the results of their successors will be met with scepticism by fans and media, who have learned the reality of what they saw in the 1990s, taken it at face value and have no wish to be deceived again.

The judiciary in France, Belgium, Holland, Switzerland and Italy have spread their net wide. French investigations have reached deep down into the ranks of amateur cyclists, touched virtually every team in the country, and, this year, went up as high as the double Tour de France winner Lance Armstrong's United States Postal Service team – against whom the allegations of malpractice remain unproven and vehemently denied at the time of writing.

After the marathon investigation sparked off by Voet's arrest, he faced trial in Lille in October 2000 with the Festina manager Bruno Roussel, PR manager Joël Chabiron and Richard Virenque. Team doctor Erik Rijckaert was absent due to illness; sadly, he died of lung cancer in late January 2001. Virenque's confession that he had indeed used EPO, entirely contrary to the version of events he had given all through the Festina inquiry, led to a tearful courtroom reconciliation with his former *soigneur*.

It also enabled him to avoid a criminal prosecution, although it earned him a ban from racing, while Voet, Roussel and Chabiron all received suspended prison sentences and fines related to supplying and inciting the use of drugs. The trial further confirmed the extent of cycling's drug problem. Indeed, the verdicts were purposely lenient, said the presiding judge Daniel Delegove, because Festina was not an isolated case.

In Italy, if anything, the inquiries have been even more extensive, following the headline-grabbing morning in June 1999 when their top cyclist Marco Pantani was rumbled. Pantani, the winner, ironically, of the stricken 1998 Tour de France, was found to have blood far thicker than the UCI's limit (a possible sign of EPO use) and was thrown off the Giro d'Italia 24 hours from the finish, when his victory had seemed assured.

In an unprecedented case, Pantani was found guilty of 'sporting fraud' for his alleged use of EPO, while a string of the greatest Italian cyclists of the 1990s have been named as receiving drugs during police inquiries into virtually every Italian trainer, including the once-legendary Michele Ferrari, and Francesco Conconi – the man paid by the International Olympic Committee to find a test for EPO.

Nearly three years post-Festina, the signs of progress

towards a cleaner sport remain mixed. Team helpers such as Voet are now licensed, and have to be properly qualified. Cyclists undergo regular, stringent medical tests to detect any signs of deteriorating health that may be caused by drug use. A test for EPO was used in the Sydney Olympics, and there were hints that this would be more widely adopted.

And yet . . . Three cyclists were thrown off the 2000 Tour before it had even begun, when they failed the blood test. The avowedly anti-drug cyclist Christophe Bassons was ostracised by his peers and quit the 1999 race a nervous wreck. And there were signs at the end of 2000 that some of the Tour's corporate backers – Fiat, Coca-Cola, Credit Lyonnais – were getting restive.

Events have moved on since *Breaking the Chain* was published in France in May 1999. But Voet's inside view of the ways of cycling leading up to the scandal remains vitally important if we are to understand the pressures which lead sportsmen to take drugs, the lies they tell themselves to justify their drug-taking, and the way in which drug-taking makes a nonsense of the notion of a level sporting playing field.

The arrest of a *soigneur* on a quiet back road on the Franco–Belgian border has already shaken the sport to its foundations: cycling will never be the same again. *Breaking the Chain* is part of a process of change which, it is to be hoped, will lead to a cleaner sport: who knows, however, if the links of the chain can be put back together again?

W.F.
London
January 2001

PREFACE

It was not an easy decision to make. Writing a book which tells the truth about the lies in cycling, going through thirty years of silence with a fine-tooth comb, testifying to the reality behind a theatrical spectacle in which I played my part for a long time; believe me, none of this was easy. And now I can expect the sarcastic epithets: the man who shattered dreams, who spat in the soup, who flung mud at a sport of the people. Fair enough: that's how you can see this if you want to pretend nothing is going on, as long as the wheels keep turning. But at what price?

What you are about to read is not motivated by bitterness or a desire for revenge. I am not passing on rumours picked up here and there, but real events which I have lived through. I have been kicking around the world of top-level cycling since 1972; as they say, I have been there, and, modest as I am, eight times out of ten I can recognise who is 'charging' and who isn't. There are little signs, which most people can't pick up.

I don't expect to make many friends with this book, which is honest, but disturbing, and will be shocking to some. There are people who have given me a good deal of support in recent months, but others, who have preferred to keep quiet without worrying too much, have simply dropped me in it. And there are those who do not want to examine their consciences, eye to eye. Because they are afraid, or because their interests are threatened? Either way, I am sorry for them.

It has not been easy to reveal these practices, which are not nice to look at. And there was a great deal to hide. Nor has it been easy stripping myself naked and putting what is left on public view. For you, the public, are involved as well because your enthusiasm and credulity have been abused. Often, I've wondered why I should be the one to come clean. Have I the right to do what no one has done before me? Who am I to reveal the poisonous secrets of a family who all have such sweet smiles in the photo album? Can I take responsibility for breaking the law of silence? Would I have produced this book if, on 8 July 1998, I had not been stopped by customs officers? I have thought long and hard and I hesitated before writing it all down. I recognise that without my time in detention, without the sixteen days I spent in prison, I would never have understood. Habit, routine and comfort have their own power. So I have done what I had to do, even if myths are shattered, even if it causes pain.

Because those who, like me, love cycling above all else no longer have a place in this arms race, with forbidden weapons, with no end in prospect. Because I feel that cycling has gone too far, leaving its original values by the roadside, and that it has no desire to make a U-turn. Because it is high time that we all understood our mistakes in order to recognise this evil, and, I hope, eradicate it. Because I felt the need to explain myself to those who are closest to me, to prove that I wasn't the bandit some people said I was. So that my children can reply to the comments, the insults. Because, in the end, someone had to do it.

Without malice, without being prudish, without making any concessions. Not by skimming the surface of this polluted world, like Erwan Mentheour, who only spent four years in the world of professional cycling and therefore was only able to produce a limited account, but by immersing myself deeply in and reviewing all the different epochs of drug-taking. Because when I was sacked without any explanation from the team where I lived out my passion for cycling, and when I was forbidden to do my job for three years – which is for ever at my age – I was turned into the perfect sacrificial lamb, the stage of the rocket which is detached to prevent the explosion, an embarrassment, a pariah. It was so easy for them. Because there are Willy Voets everywhere. The difference is that I decided to step out of line.

I am fifty-four. I have lost my job, my health is bad, I can't sleep without sleeping pills and my nights are no longer peaceful. But for all this, I still have my dreams. Like that of seeing my son Mathieu talk to me about cycling with the gleam in his eyes he used to have. I have been awaiting trial for a year, but, in spite of how it might appear, I have become a free man. I have more freedom, at any rate, than those who ride bearing this banner, which is very hard to carry.

This is why.

Veynes
April 1999

ONE

CHAMPAGNE, DRIPS AND MY WIFE'S FRIDGE

I may be Belgian, but the French national championship is the one race which I really loved to go to when I was working at Festina. It was one of the few opportunities I used to get to take along my wife Sylvie and two of my children as guests of the sponsor. When I was on the road for more than 200 days a year, that weekend together at the end of June or in early July meant a lot.

It was 4 July 1998, the day before the championship. We left our flat in Veynes, in the Hautes Alpes, at about seven a.m. I was on the way to meet my extended family, taking my own small family in the Renault 21. Sylvie was at the wheel. In December 1997, after being caught speeding for the fourth time, my licence had been taken away for six months, so I had to be driven. Still I enjoyed the trip up to Clermont Ferrand, with Mathieu and Charlotte in the back, because it was my birthday. I was fifty-three years old and I'd hardly noticed the time passing.

We arrived at the Inter Hotel at about eleven-thirty. Waiting for the cyclists to come in from training, I killed time talking to the mechanics, Cyrille Perrin and Patrick Jean. 'They won't be long, they're only going out for a couple of hours.'

In fact, the first group wasted no time in coming back: Pascal Hervé, Christophe Moreau, Laurent Brochard, Didier Rous and Richard Virenque, the French riders who were going to start the Tour de France.

'Where are the others?'

'They're on their way, they're coming.'

Most of the time the team split into two distinct groups. On one side there were the riders who were going to race the Tour, the strong men who could race hard no matter what the weather. On the other was the rest of the team: Christophe Bassons, Patrice Halgand, young Laurent Lefevre, Sebastian Médan, and Thierry Laurent, riders who were not involved in the drug-taking that was later to mar their team mates' careers. They even ate as two little groups in the evening. I was used to this by now, but it shocked my wife. 'Good to see they all stick together,' she murmured in my ear.

I introduced Sylvie and the children to the riders who were new that season, unloaded the car, and then set up my massage table. I gave Virenque, Brochard and Rous their rub-downs just after lunch, we spent a quiet afternoon and then went down for dinner.

That evening the team gathered around four tables in the main room of the restaurant: at one table were the Tour team and their wives; at the next, the other cyclists with their partners; at the third, the masseurs and mechanics; at the fourth, the management – Bruno Roussel, the team manager, his deputy Michel Gros, and Joël Chabiron, the PR man, all with their wives. This was the way we usually divided up throughout the year, depending on what tables there were in the restaurants.

I ordered champagne. It might have been the day before a major race, but you have to celebrate your birthday. Three bottles to drink with our desserts. The waiter brought the cake, a black forest gâteau ordered by Bruno Roussel. At their tables, the riders lifted their flutes and toasted me, singing. Pascal Hervé and Richard Virenque even came over to give me a hug and wish me happy birthday.

After dinner I went to get the *bidons* – plastic bottles

which mount on the bikes – ready for the race, with another *soigneur*, Laurent Gros, Michel's son. Usually we put water and syrup or energy drink in them. Then we got the food ready to hand up to the riders the next day. Finally, at about ten o'clock, I went up to my room. Usually I do it in the riders' rooms, but it was out of the question in front of their wives.

'It'? An intramuscular injection of cortisone for each of them, Hervé, Virenque, Brochard, Rous and Moreau, ten milligrammes of Kenacort in one buttock. It can't be detected in the urine. In the case of a blood test, the doctor can ascertain that there is an abnormality, but cannot be certain that the cortisone is exogenous because the suprarenal glands produce it naturally. This is one of the reasons why the riders who 'charge up' swear that they don't take drugs. They actually believe what they say! Simply because the substances don't show up at the doping controls. Out of sight, out of mind.

The effect of corticoids is perverse: they are natural painkillers produced by the adrenal glands, but when they are injected the glands shut down. This is why sportspeople who abuse them can end up with deficiencies, notably of calcium; their immune systems are weakened too. If they break a bone, the fracture can take an immensely long time to knit. Prolonged use of cortisone is therefore utter madness; but that was the last thing I worried about, nor was I concerned about the caravan where the riders would deliver urine samples for testing after the finish at Charade. The only question I asked myself was about the correct dose to inject. So close to the Tour de France, you have to use the bare minimum of cortisone because of its effect on the immune system, which is placed under such extreme pressure during the Tour. The effects, muscle pain relief, are felt immediately after the injection and rise quickly for six hours until reaching *une pointe*, a peak, after which they rapidly fall away again.

3

★ ★ ★

With the injections out of the way, I checked each rider's haematocrit, the level of solid matter in the blood. This is a rough indicator of the level of red cells, which carry oxygen to the muscles. For an endurance athlete, such as a cyclist, the higher this level is the better – but only as long as it's safe. Brochard was at 47, Rous at 49.7, Virenque at 50.2. Pascal Hervé was right up to 51.3, while Christophe Moreau was bang on 48. A healthy man in his twenties would usually be between 41 and 44, but such unnaturally high figures were just what we expected.

We were just a week away from the start of the Tour de France. Approaching the team's biggest objective of the season, the level had to be as close as possible to the upper limit of 50, which cycling's governing body, the Union Cycliste Internationale (UCI), judged to be safe for a rider's health. During the race all that remained to be done was to keep it at that level. But if a rider was at 45 per cent beforehand, for example, it would be impossible to raise the level during the race because the rider is under too much physical stress. But aside from the Tour, the national championship was a big race and the riders wanted to win, Virenque especially. It was on a particularly tough course and was his first real test of the year.

Just in case the UCI doctors arrived in the morning to check the riders' haematocrit levels, I got everything ready to get them through the tests. We were so used to doing this that there was nothing out of the ordinary about it. I went up to the cyclists' rooms with sodium drips, flasks of water mixed with 0.09 per cent sodium. As a precaution, I wrapped them in a towel before sliding them under the beds. In an emergency, you just had to take a picture off the wall and use the hook to hang the drip from. If there was no picture hook, I took a bicycle wheel spoke, bent it into an S and hung it from something else, like a curtain rail.

The rest was child's play: put the tap into the drip, stick the needle into the rider's arm, open the tap and check the first few drips – no more than sixty a minute to avoid any shock to the system. After that I would open the tap fully because there was no danger. The whole transfusion would take twenty minutes, the saline diluting the blood and so reducing the haematocrit level by three units – just enough.

This contraption took no more than two minutes to set up, which meant we could put it into action while the UCI doctors waited for the riders to come down from their rooms. Bruno Roussel would be told first that the doctors were coming, and then they would come to my room and that of the team doctor, Eric Rijckaert, if he was on the road with us. And off we went . . .

When the first haematocrit level tests were carried out on the Paris–Nice in March 1997, we had been ready since the winter or, more precisely, since the UCI had announced that it was bringing the tests in. At first, I was the only person to have the battery-operated machine for testing the haematocrit level, which we called the 'centrifuge' and which Rijckaert had bought in Germany. It was worth over 3,000 francs, and the riders were queuing up to use it in my room! But after the 1997 Tour de France, the checks became more widespread, and by 1998 about two-thirds of the riders had their own machines. They had bought them by mail order, using the name of their wife or daughter when placing the order. You can't be too careful.

This little magic box, 20 centimetres by 8, is an invaluable tool. We used to take the blood sample straight out of the artery, which was more accurate than putting a needle into a fingertip because the blood is more concentrated. For each rider, we would fill two short tubes, which were thinner than a ballpoint refill. It only took a few drops, less than a centilitre. The tubes would be slipped into the centrifuge, which turns at 10,000 revolutions per minute for about two minutes, before stopping automatically. When you open the centrifuge, the plasma, which is the colour of egg white, has separated from the red cells. It only remains to read the haematocrit level on the scale – it's the dividing line between the red cells and the plasma. To be extra precise, I used a magnifying glass. And the job was done.

Richard Virenque lost the French championship that year, and he lost it because he rode like an idiot. The circuit was made for him, he was at a peak of fitness, and it seemed to us that even Laurent Jalabert on his best form would not be able to beat him. The course, eleven laps with some steep climbs, was one which would gradually weed out the weaker riders. He just had to keep his place in the first twenty, chasing any dangerous-looking attacks and then, about two laps from the finish, when the lead group was down to the strongest riders, give it all he had.

Richard went to the start in his own car. Like everyone else, I'd tried to get through to him: 'Richard, I know you. Don't do anything, let the other riders make the running, no one can beat you,' because with him, being such an impulsive and impatient character, it was better to ram the message home. I was wasting my time! About halfway through the race a breakaway group developed, with Hervé and Brochard among them. They're among the best at moves of that kind, so Richard should have been able to sit back and let others do the work to recapture them. But of course he had to lead the chase. And as he brought the bunch back to the leaders, Jalabert counter-attacked at once with Luc Leblanc and a few others. Richard had cut his own throat. Not one Festina in front. Panic stations! Bruno Roussel went crazy and made the team chase; gradually Virenque, Hervé and a few others made it back to the front, but they had left a lot of their energy on the road. The damage was done. Au revoir, gold medal.

You can imagine the ambience when we got back to the hotel, but we had to get over the disappointment and think of the Tour. Before they left for home, I had given each rider a very special *bidon*: at the bottom were two capsules of erithropoetin (EPO) of 2,000 units each, and two small tubes of powder to mix it with, all covered in ice cubes right up to the neck. And on Sunday evening I left with my family, with Sylvie at the wheel of our car, while I drove a Festina station wagon. I know, I didn't have a licence . . .

On Monday morning, I had a call from Dr Rijckaert, who wanted me to drive to his home in Ghent the next day to pick up ten boxes of drips. In France, one–litre drips are sold in glass containers, which aren't convenient to move around or get rid of. It's better to use plastic ones. So I set off on Tuesday at eight a.m.

Behind my seat were two refrigerated bags, one red, one blue. They contained 234 doses of EPO, 80 flasks of human growth hormone, 160 capsules of male hormone, testosterone, and 60 pills called Asaflow, a product based on aspirin, which makes the blood more fluid. This whole chemical works had been stored in my house for the previous month in the vegetable basket of our fridge, which had not gone down too well with my wife, not so much because she had no idea where to put the carrots, but because she doubted that the stuff was harmless.

A few weeks earlier, on 1 June, I had driven to the car park of the Buffalo Grill, near Bordeaux's Merignac airport, at about seven o'clock. Using my mobile phone, I'd arranged the meeting point as we drove. I had hired a car, a metallic blue Peugeot 306, so as not to be noticed (a Festina team car can be spotted at ten kilometres!). Carine, my daughter from my first marriage, was driving. I had come to pick up the magic potions, although Carine knew nothing

7

about that. I made the trip twice a year, in February and June.

We were waiting for Joël Chabiron, the team's PR man, who was coming from Portugal with his car loaded up. As he was late, Carine and I had dinner. At last he arrived, at the wheel of his Mercedes, with a couple whom I didn't recognise. It was the foulest weather ever. In sheets of rain, we parked bumper to bumper. Chabiron had the stuff in the bottom of the boot, in a big sports bag covered with clothes. We took it all out and transferred it straight to the refrigerated bags. A quick handshake and we parted.

On the road to Ghent in July, I stopped off at Meyzieu, where the team has its logistics base. I made sure that nothing was missing from the lorry, which was about to set off for Ireland and the start of the Tour on the following Saturday. I left my suitcase, keeping with me the drugs, my briefcase and a black rucksack, which contained everything I needed for a day. I took a Festina estate car to Evry, in the Paris suburbs, to pick up an official car from the Tour de France organisers and from there I went on to Rijckaert's house in Zomergem, arriving early in the evening.

Eric offered me dinner, but I had arranged to meet a good friend in Brussels. Off I went, with the drips and drugs in the boot. Next morning I was to get a boat from Calais, before driving across England to Dublin. Easy as one-two-three.

TWO
ANYTHING TO DECLARE?

That Wednesday, I was up at five-thirty a.m. After a quick wash, I was behind the wheel bang on six o'clock, without even shaving. As I hadn't had much sleep, I had taken a 'taster' to help me keep going: an injection of 'Belgian mix'. It came in a tiny little bottle, 10, 15 or sometimes 20 millilitres of a clear liquid, which you injected after pricking the rubber top with a needle. Back then, I didn't have any real notion of what the flask contained, beyond amphetamines, which were what I wanted. It was two months later that a television journalist let me know the exact contents of this cocktail. In alphabetical order they were amphetamines, caffeine, cocaine, heroin, painkillers and sometimes corticosteroids: a magic potion to keep you up all night.

It's no more than three hours' drive from Brussels to Calais, so I had plenty of time. There were two options: go through Valenciennes and take the turn-off for Calais, or go back towards Ghent and Kortrijk on the E17 motorway towards Lille. To this day I don't quite know why I went for this route. Coming up to the border – and I still don't know why I did this either – I decided to fork right. The day before Rijckaert had told me to be careful, so perhaps that's why I decided to leave the motorway at the very last minute. I learned later that the back road I took is used by small-time drug-dealers.

It was about a quarter to seven. I was going down the little French road without a care in the world when I spotted a man standing at the roadside a hundred metres ahead of me. As I drew nearer, I realised he was a customs officer. My heart began beating like a drum. It was too late for a U-turn. When I was level with him, the customs man signalled to me to pull over. I didn't know what to do. It was the first time in over thirty years' driving that I had been stopped. It was just my luck. As I pulled up, I saw the white van parked in the bushes. And then everything happened very quickly. Four customs men got out of the van and surrounded the car.

In actual fact, if I was quaking in my boots, it wasn't because of what I was carrying behind my car seat, but because of the Belgian mix. And not just the little jar that I'd injected from, but another one, which was destined for Laurent Dufaux. Three months earlier, in the finish area of the Flèche Wallonne one-day Classic, I had met up with an old friend, a former professional, who was wearing a race pass. While we were waiting for the riders to reach the finish – and they were a good hour away – we talked about the weather, but then he offered to barter two pots of Belgian mix for a Festina team-issue jersey, a pair of shorts and a pair of cycling tights. We clinched the deal a little way away, in front of a house where the riders would be getting changed. I had to filch the clothing from the riders' bags and replace the missing items from the stock in the team lorry when we got back to the hotel.

One of the two bottles was for me. When you're driving more than 130,000 kilometres a year, you have to stay awake. The riders take drugs – but so do those who look after them. I'd rather take 10 milligrammes of amphetamines than wrap my car round a plane tree. As for Dufaux, I had bought a Yorkshire terrier from him at Christmas for my daughter Charlotte. It was worth 4,000 francs, and I'd paid him only 3,000 francs. Dufaux had said that if I could find him a flask of Belgian mix, he'd forget the rest. My friend's offer had come at just the right time . . . The flasks usually contain 15 millilitres; depending on how much you want to take, that works out at about 15 injections of one millilitre. You can keep going for the whole season on just one pot. Hit the jackpot the whole year round.

So that's why, three months later, I had two flasks of Belgian mix stuffed into my rucksack on the passenger seat. I didn't even think about the EPO. I grabbed the two flasks and just had time to stuff one into my right trouser pocket. The other one was still in my hand when a customs man appeared at the window and asked if I had anything to declare. Good question. I just answered, 'Oh, not really, just vitamins for the riders.' He didn't even ask me to show my papers, just to open the boot. I hoped I'd be able to slip the flasks into one of the cool bags, but they didn't take their eyes off me for a second. As I lifted up the boot lid, I threw the pot I was holding into the bushes. The other one was still stuffed in my pocket.

To show willing, I moved one of the boxes of drips, but one of the customs men made a sign at me to show that it was pointless. I thought everything was going fine, that I had no reason to get alarmed, but while this was going on his colleagues had come across the two cool bags behind the passenger seat. They opened them, took out the Tupperware cartons covered in frozen bottles of water and asked me what was in them. 'Erm, I don't know. Stuff to help the riders recover, I think.'

'Well, if you don't know, you're coming with us.'

The name of the place where they caught me, I found out later, was Dronckaert – Flemish for alcoholic. And I hardly ever drink even a glass of wine. With a customs man sitting

11

next to me in the car, I followed the van to the customs post, about a kilometre away. I was strung up like a violin and my passenger was trying to make me calm down. He kept talking to me about the Tour, which was about to start, about Virenque's form . . . I could hardly hear what he was going on about. I was saying to myself, 'You're dead meat, Willy my boy. Kaput. Finished. Curtains.' I thought of the pot of Belgian mix stuffed in my pocket and the cool bags, which were ahead of me in the van. No chance of getting them back now. And me, the idiot, caught at the border carrying drugs. A catastrophe. But I had no inkling of what was actually going to happen.

The heavy gate opened automatically into a large red–brick building. The van parked in front of it and my passenger made a sign to me to keep going. When I saw in my mirror that the gate was closing behind me, I began to have difficulty breathing. When we came to a stop I wanted to pick up my rucksack, but the customs man wouldn't let me.

'Don't touch anything.'

I followed him, while his colleagues took care of my car. They went through everything. From the upholstery on the doors to the screen wash, from the elbow rest to the indicators. Everything. Looking through the windows of the building, I watched the whole show. Then I was taken into an office.

One of the three customs men began emptying the contents of the cool bags on to a table. I was so thirsty that I asked if I could have one of the bottles of water and swigged half of it in one go. Methodically, they placed the capsules on the table, lining them up like model soldiers. I looked at my watch: time was passing. I was meant to be on the ten o'clock boat from Calais. That Belgian mix was in my pocket.

'Excuse me, but is this going to take long? I've got a boat to catch.'

'You can forget about the boat.'

They continued making an inventory of the stuff. When one of the customs men recorded a capsule of EPO and a tube of powder as two doses, I tried to explain that the two together made one dose, but he didn't want to know. And he just went on counting the tubes of powder . . . The capsules of EPO with red lids were lined up in one row and the little flasks of human growth hormone with their blue covers were lined up next to them. All the little flasks were sealed with a large label written out in Spanish or Portuguese. On the other side of the table was a line of 'Easter eggs', which is what we used to call the brown balls of testosterone. The riders knew what I was talking about when I offered them Easter eggs. Always taken orally, testosterone was undetectable, although a positive test was possible if it was injected into the muscle.

Continuing with their work, the customs men kept asking me what everything was, to which I invariably gave the same answer: 'I don't know.' In the end, as I didn't change my tune, one of them announced that they would have the stuff tested by a laboratory in Lille. Then, having emptied my rucksack and briefcase without missing anything, they took me into another, larger office, where an older, more relaxed-looking officer was sitting. I found out later that he was just a few days off retirement. He gave me a newspaper, discussed the World Cup, which was at its height, and even offered me a cup of coffee. Until then I had been dealing with rather cold, distant officials, who no doubt took me for a drug-dealer. But he made me feel a little bit more human. I relaxed slightly.

'Ah, if only I'd known, I'd have gone the other way. I'd be coming into Calais about now.'

'If we hadn't picked you up here, we'd have got you there anyway.'

I tried to find out more, but he wouldn't go into details. I could feel he was a bit embarrassed, as if he'd said too much. He kept talking about this and that. He was a nice guy, perhaps too nice. I needed some peace and quiet. I buried myself in a book, more to cut myself off from everything than because I wanted to read. And then there was the smell in the air, the characteristic whiff of somewhere where life goes on in slow motion . . .

Another customs officer appeared at the door.

'Monsieur, as this is a serious matter, we will have to have you body-searched.'

I was stunned. With what I had in my pocket, I was done for. However, he disappeared for a few moments, and while the older customs officer was doing something with the coffee machine I managed to slide the flask into my underpants.

I had never been in a situation like this before and I still thought I would be able to wriggle my way out somehow. When the man came back, I had to get undressed. I was not wearing much as it was the beginning of July. First I took off my white polo shirt, a Festina team-issue one, which the customs man inspected carefully.

'Shoes.'

I took off my shoes, which he examined closely, trying to pull the heels apart.

'Trousers.'

He took them, held them upside down and turned the pockets inside out.

'Socks.'

I handed them over at arm's length.

'Now your underpants.'

I'd thought he wasn't going to ask for them. I waited a moment.

'Underpants, please.'

I wanted to buy some time, scratched my nose, the back of my neck, sniffed, but, in the end I had to take my underpants off, slowly, with my legs clasped together so that the Belgian mix remained stuck under my testicles. Just like a stripper. Finally, I gave him the underpants.

'Open your legs. Come on, open your legs!'

It was the end of the road. Ping! The pot hit the floor. And I did too. About now, the boat was sailing out of Calais without me.

I thought the customs officer was going to lose it. With one of his colleagues helping, he forced me into a chair and handcuffed my left wrist to a ring in the wall. A doctor turned up, wearing jeans and a shirt. He put on a surgical glove and slipped a finger up my anus.

'You're going to hospital for X-rays.'

It was as if I'd been sandbagged. Suddenly, I'd stopped being a masseur and had become a drug-dealer. I was being taken for something I wasn't. What had I done that they should treat me like this?

I put my clothes back on, and was taken to the hospital. On the way we passed my disembowelled car, which was being photographed. It looked as if it had been through much the same experience as I had. After the X-ray, which of course showed nothing, I was taken back to the customs office. My fate would only be known when the results of the analyses came through. I waited for hours, handcuffed again, while a few metres away the customs officers were discussing their gardens and what was on the telly. They were getting on with their lives while I had just passed through the gates of hell.

During the afternoon, a customs man in plain clothes, a big guy, burst in. He began calling me names and got seriously heavy with me.

'This is going right to the top. You're all going to pay dearly for this, Festina's sunk.'

He obviously wanted to intimidate me, make me crack. I didn't have any spirit for the fight. The less I told him, the more annoyed he became. He really disturbed me, and he was the one who took down my first statement. I told him I didn't understand why where the stuff came from mattered. As far as I was concerned, I'd taken whatever it was out of my fridge, got into the car and started driving. Then when I hit the border all this started. They didn't believe a word I was saying, they clearly thought I was a trafficker. And there was this young customs man with the nasty, disbelieving look, banging his fist on the table. I thought his next punch was coming at me. Actually, intimidation was his style and nothing more, but I hadn't worked that out yet and he scared me. Throughout the affair, this was the only official who really made me sick. The others were just doing what they had to do.

After the interrogation, at about five o'clock, I ended up back in the office of the old customs man. Again he made me a coffee, offered me a sandwich. I hadn't eaten since the previous evening, but I wasn't exactly starving. I asked him if I could call my wife, but he refused in no uncertain terms.

'I'll use my mobile. Bring it in, it's in the car.'

'Are you taking the piss?'

Constantly handcuffed, never left alone, I sat on my chair. The results of the analyses came in at about eight o'clock: EPO, growth hormone, testosterone.

'Really? I guess it could be. I don't know anything about it. If you say so, I'll believe you.'

In the next-door office, they called the police. The one who seemed to be the boss came over. 'At ten, you're going to the "central" in Lille.'

Two of the customs men who had arrested me that morning were still with me. They'd had a long day, and it was all down to me. So they took me into the rooms set aside for down time in the building next door. It was the France–Croatia match that evening, a World Cup quarter final which they weren't going to miss for anything. Zidane and the players of the French team helped to lighten the atmosphere. Before kick-off, the three customs men began asking me about cycling. Were all the riders on drugs? What about footballers, were they as well? Just everyday questions, and, to round it all off, two goals from Thuram! During the match one of them even offered me something to eat.

'What would you say to a plate of chips?'

What wouldn't I have said?

'Spot of mayonnaise?'

I'd have taken chilli sauce, I was so hungry.

'Ham or sausage?'

I was coming back to life. No handcuffs. The smell of coffee, chips. It was as if a bit of home was being rebuilt around me. I went for the sausage. What a shame we had to get ready to go at quarter to ten. One last glance at the television and the two customs men drove me down to the 'central', the seat of Lille's police department, the SRPJ.

They put the handcuffs back on as we got out of the van. It was the rules. Then they left me for a while, sitting on a bench and handcuffed to the wall, in a never-ending corridor. On one side was a long row of cells. Not an attractive prospect. In front of the bars was a plate of transparent plastic, meant to hide the misery kept inside, but it couldn't hide the voices. Everywhere, there was shouting, insults, swear words. Suddenly a man in handcuffs sprang out of nowhere, dragged by two cops, yelling at the end of the corridor. He was struggling so much that the policemen pushed him to the ground. He began kicking them, but their response was harsh. Another cop turned up and they laid into him. All this just to reach the same final result: bunged in a cell.

When I ended up on the first floor, in an office, in front of the officer who was on guard duty that night, I could only think about keeping my nose clean. One formality followed another. I had to confirm my name, my age, my height, my place of residence, my state of health, the name of my mother . . . And I wondered what she, who had been dead for a quarter of a century, would have made of all this.

'Two officers from the justice department will come and collect you tomorrow at eight o'clock. While you're waiting, you'll be put in a cell.'

I went back down. I was made to take off my belt, my laces and even my glasses before I was taken into the cell, into which three scruffily dressed men and a woman had already been squeezed. The stench was indescribable. Puke, booze, urine, farts, shit, all mixed together. I was going to have to spend an entire night in this hole and try to keep the tears back. I curled up on the end of a bench, hugging my knees, my back glued to the wall. I forced my eyelids down. From time to time I could hear my cellmates groaning, asking to be let out to go to the toilet, then pissing in a corner. My eyes were closed, but I didn't get any sleep that night, the most desperate night of my life.

THREE

NUMBER 237, AT THE END ON THE LEFT

It was a relief when the gendarmes came to get me half an hour early the following morning. There were two of them, one with a thin moustache and glasses, the other one well fed to say the least: Jean-Marie and Robert. They were waiting in the hall, where I got my rucksack back. According to the rule book, they should have handcuffed me before putting me in the official grey Peugeot 405 waiting in the yard.

'Come on, you're not going to run off, are you?'

All Robert did before setting off was make sure that the back doors were locked. He got his cigarettes out as soon as we left the 'central'.

'Fancy one?'

Back then, I'd only smoked about ten a day, but I hadn't had one since Tuesday evening. That fag was a taste of freedom!

It was rush hour. Robert lost his patience.

'Get your contraption out, Jean-Marie.' He rummaged under the seat, pulled down the window and stuck the blue flashing light on the roof. Everyone got out of the way until we reached an ordinary-looking gate, like a garage door, which Jean-Marie opened with a remote control. We went into a huge car park.

'Bring your bag and come with us.'

At the lift door we bumped into the 'boss', who seemed

to know who I was. Then we went up to the office which Jean-Marie and Robert shared.

'First of all, let's have a nice cup of coffee,' said Jean-Marie. 'Do you want one, Willy? What do you reckon?'

Robert added, 'And I'm going to pop out to the *boulangerie*. Croissant or pain au chocolat, Willy?'

Coffee and pastries – I thought I was dreaming. After breakfast, they sat down in front of their computer. They had my statements, my rucksack, my briefcase and the two cool bags, which had still not been resealed. And they began to question me, reading through what I'd said the day before. Just to check. It was all friendly until, abruptly, Jean-Marie cut through the gentle chit-chat.

'Do you really take us for dickheads?'

I said nothing.

'Do you stand by these statements, sir?' This time the intimate tone had gone.

'Er, yes.'

So they shifted to another method of interrogation: asking the same questions again and again in different ways, in a more and more aggressive tone. I felt myself shrinking down into my seat. To avoid being overwhelmed I asked if I could call Sylvie.

'As long as you refuse to co-operate, we can't allow it. And how do we know you won't talk in a secret code?'

Jean-Marie went out. Robert waited for a second before going on.

'Listen, Willy, don't you think it would be better if you just told us the truth? We'll take your statements, no worries. But everything's going to be pinned on you. Who are you scared of? Tell me. I won't take any notes, it's off the record.'

He'd gone back to being friendly.

'A few weeks ago we had a training camp in Corrèze, down near Brive, to look over the time-trial stage of the

Tour. Someone invited us to a big château because we happened to be down there. Do you know who it was? Bernadette Chirac. Virenque and Brochard were there — that's how important those guys are. That's what I'm scared of. It's a lot bigger than Willy Voet. Do you see?'

'Hold on. Do you know whose backside was on the chair you're sitting on now a few months ago? Bernard Tapie's. And we squashed him like a fly. Your Virenque and your Brochard don't mean a thing to us. You'd better think it over. If you want five years inside, that's your problem. We'll just take down the statement and that's it, job done. But think about your wife and kids. Because the people you're trying to protect won't look after them when you've been banged up, I can tell you.'

Jean-Marie came back, and after talking a little, they agreed that I could call Sylvie. Jean-Marie dialled the number.

'Good morning, madame. This is the SRPJ in Lille. Your husband is with us. We can't divulge any information to do with the matter which is keeping him here, both for his own safety and for official reasons to do with our enquiries. You may speak to him, but you may not ask him anything. He will talk to you merely in order to tell you that he's fit and well. But not a single question, agreed?'

Of course my wife's first sentence was a question: 'What on earth's going on?'

'Nothing, nothing, don't worry. Don't ask any questions. I'm fine. How are the children? Are you all right?'

Then Sylvie asked another question, the obvious one, which to her seemed quite innocuous. 'Does Bruno Roussel know where you are?'

It was the breakthrough they'd been waiting for. All that was in her mind was whether my employer ought to know what had happened, but the police assumed she was talking about a drug deal.

'Madame, you have been requested not to ask any questions. I apologise, but we must end this conversation at once.'

It was getting on for lunchtime. They put me in the cell next door with a sandwich in my hands. As he locked the door, Robert just whispered, 'Have a good think, Willy. We'll be back about two o'clock. Think long and hard.'

After they came back, it all started again.

'Right, what was that question about? Why did your wife ask you if Bruno Roussel knows where you are?'

There was no point in holding out any longer. Drop by painful drop, they would have wrung the truth out of me. I thought of Sylvie, Charlotte and Mathieu, and began to confess everything. I began by going through the part played by Bruno Roussel and Eric Rijckaert, but I still tried to protect some of the other team members, Joël Chabiron for example.

So how had I come by the drugs?

'They were brought in from Spain in the team lorry. The doctors just ask us to carry them. They are the ones who put in the orders, or at least I think so, I don't really know much about it . . .'

I was saying anything that came into my head, and every time they came back at me I just got more bogged down. It was pathetic. Each time they asked a new question I was trapped. After typing in my new, incomplete statement, they wanted to take some time off.

'Right, you're going back to the "central" for the night. Tomorrow we'll do a bit more, and you can go in front of the investigating judge.'

No, please, not the 'central'. The very thought of going back there turned my stomach. I asked them to do me a favour: anywhere, as long as it wasn't there, please. They were a bit reluctant, then called a small police station out in the suburbs. Phew, there was some space. The station was clean – almost luxurious in comparison with the previous night. Three cells and just one guy in custody, me. The gendarme on duty gave me two blankets against the cold. He even let me hang on to my glasses. It was only a plank bench, but I could sleep, at last.

Friday, 10 July, seven-thirty a.m. Same actors, same script. Jean-Marie, Robert, the blue flashing light, the police station. After yet more questions, they took my fingerprints. It was a strange feeling. And they took my picture, which was even more humiliating. A portrait with a card in my hand, then side-on. So I was a criminal – just thinking about it makes me want to cry even now. About that time, they told me that my period of detention had been extended so that they could question me further.

Around nine o'clock we set off for the Palais de Justice. The 405 parked near the 'mousehole', an underground entry at the back of the building. I was made to wait in a large cell with about twenty other prisoners. We were allowed to smoke, so I had a fag. That morning, Robert had beckoned to me. 'Here, have these,' he muttered, passing me a packet of cigarettes.

All around me, everyone was telling their hard-luck stories. One guy had given his girlfriend a belting because he'd found her astride the guy from across the landing; another one had ripped off a load of washing machines; someone else had nicked a lorryload of potatoes to sell them on in Belgium . . . And me? I'd been transporting another kind of gear. These little confidences shared, I left my fellow criminals to go to the judge's office on the tenth floor, together with my two guardian angels.

'We've got other things to do. We have to leave you here. Have a nice day.'

Amongst the 'other things' was the small matter of

searching my house the next morning, as the law required. As they left, Robert and Jean-Marie introduced me to a duty lawyer, Maître Ludovic Baron. Before being taken in to the judge, we talked for a few minutes.

'I've consulted your file. I'll try and get you out of here.'

But first the judge had to agree.

Going into the judge's office, I was dumbfounded. I had been expecting a large, impressive chamber; instead it was a tiny, square room with two desks, one for the judge and one for his stenographer.

Alongside Judge Keil, who had a serious, direct but honest look to him, was a brown-haired woman: his assistant. I went through my routine in front of them and she showed me no mercy.

'This is a shameful case. People like that, who live by cheating, should be locked up.'

The judge interrupted. 'I'm going to have to keep you in detention. For your own safety to start with, but also because of the significance of this case, which will be heavily covered by the media. I don't want you to have any contact with the outside world for the time being. You will be held in the detention centre at Loos in a separate block, where we put young offenders, a long way from the other detainees and in solitary confinement. It's better that way.'

I was both disappointed and shocked. After a quick consultation with the lawyer, I was taken down to the basement, where I ended up among prisoners who were inside on serious charges. In this huge room, a real Babel, I was kept without food or drink until eight o'clock. We had to wait for all the other detainees to go before their particular investigating judge before leaving for Loos. In the Black Maria there were fourteen of us, locked in individual compartments, seven on either side of the van. The guards held us in threes and fours on leashes, which they had passed through our handcuffs before turning the key.

Once inside the prison, the van went through three sets of wooden gates which opened and closed automatically. Of the fourteen of us, only two were new boys: Silvano, an Italian, and me. It was too late for them to put me in solitary. After filling out all the forms and handing over my personal effects, I had to spend my first night at Loos with Silvano. He was a former drug addict of about thirty who poured out his life story to me; telling me of his brother who died of an overdose, how he had mugged old people, 'but without hitting them', his fears, his way of life . . . He couldn't hold it in. You never imagine all that suffering when you live in a bubble. Silvano got on my wick, but I couldn't tell him where to get off. Since we were allowed to smoke and I didn't have any cigarettes on me, he offered me one of his roll-ups. When he licked the paper, I felt a stab of disgust. He'd been a drug addict . . . But I wanted the smoke so much.

A key ring banged along the metal bars. The wake-up call at six-thirty was brutal. First of all I went to see the prison doctor, who filled in a medical form before looking me over quickly, mainly at my arms to see if I'd been shooting up. What was hurting was my head. I'd had a violent migraine for two days – I couldn't take it any more. He took my blood pressure.

'I'm not surprised you've got a headache. Your blood pressure's way up.'

He gave me some pills straight away and I'm still taking them to this day.

From the sickbay I was taken to see the psychologist, a woman of about forty, who asked me about what had led me to be where I was today, and about what I'd like to do when I left prison. As if I had any idea what was going to become of me . . .

The news of my detention had spread throughout the prison, thanks to the television news, which was being watched in every cell. Every time I met one of the guards, or even other prisoners, who were pushing food trolleys or cleaning out the showers, I could hear them saying my name, that they'd seen me 'on the box'. It has to be said that I wasn't hard to pick out, what with my prison number written in large letters on my Festina team-issue polo shirt.

At the clothing room I picked up two sheets and two blankets, two pairs of underpants, two T-shirts and stuff to eat with. They may take away your belt and laces, but they give you a knife, a fork, a spoon and two disposable razors. The person who was handing out all these things recognised me as well.

'You're Willy Voet, aren't you? The shit's going to hit the fan now. I'm a cyclist myself, I love the whole thing.'

A guard then took me to the second floor, to D wing. He opened the door. I will never forget the number: 237, the last door but one on the left at the end of the corridor. The cell, about eight square metres of concrete, was full of dust. On the right as you went in was the toilet, which was cracked, and not exactly four-star. Then the washbasin – cold water only. At the far end on the same side was a wardrobe with four shelves but no door, while on the left was the iron bed, screwed to the wall, with a misshapen mattress. And, wonder of wonders, right up above, a brand-new, shining colour television. Home sweet home.

Finally, on the back wall, was a large rectangular window with two shutters and six bars, through which you could just make out the sky. To see a little more, I had to climb on a central heating pipe which ran across the cell. I could see the yard, where twice a day the prisoners were allowed to exercise, once in the morning, once in the afternoon. On the right, behind some buildings, I could hear canal barges. As a kid I had lived near a canal and the familiar sound of the motors made me homesick. In prison the slightest thing takes you back, as if your thoughts are reflected in a mirror.

So there I was. I was about to begin two weeks' rest cure. Harder to cope with than the threats of the young plain clothes customs officer, tougher than the living nightmare of the 'central', was the icy finger of fear that ran down my back, until the silence seemed to suffocate, filling my guts, my ears, my heart, to the depth of my soul. This feeling gnawed away at me, this fear of emptiness and then nothing more. I wouldn't wish it on my worst enemy.

I cried as I had never cried before.

FOUR

I WILL SURVIVE

I can't remember how long I spent just lying there. After the warder found me some cleaning stuff and I'd cleared out the cell (I'll never say 'my cell'), I spent almost the whole weekend asleep. I wasn't even bothered by the constant noise of the prisoners yelling their frustration, the curses they kept screaming.

Saturday 11 July was a beautiful day. Pressing up against the bars, I could see the prisoners out enjoying themselves in the yard. Some were playing football, some were just chatting. On one side a couple of guys were sitting with their heads in their hands. I thought of my wife. She would never find better grounds for divorce. I thought of my children. How would they take it? And their schoolfriends, the neighbours, the rest of the family? My in-laws in particular, because my parents had passed away and my only brother had died when I was ten.

A good wash, that would make me think of something else. For four days I hadn't washed or shaved. I had not had a change of clothes either: I was disgusting and was duly disgusted. What a joy the cold water was . . . Shaving with soap – so sweet. Then I switched the television on. There was nothing else to do. Ponder and weep, sleep and have nightmares, watch the box. It was the day of the opening time trial of the Tour de France, the great send-off, the beginning of the festival. On the podium in Dublin, during the team presentation, I even saw the Festina riders file past one by one. They didn't look too happy with life – as if they could sense that the boomerang was about to fly back in their faces.

When I heard the food trolley, I reckoned that lunchtime must have come. It was a quarter to twelve. Served up by one of the prisoners, the menu was spartan: a big spoonful of baked beans, two sausages, a yoghurt and fresh or stewed fruit. As I was a newcomer, the server passed me two baguettes – 'That's for two days' – some sugar and four squares of butter for the next morning's breakfast. Thirty seconds of contact with the outside world.

The first visitor was the chaplain. I'm not much of a one for Mass. If you're into that you end up being late for the Tour of Flanders or Paris–Roubaix or some other big race on a Sunday. But his arrival was comforting. He was kind and plain-speaking. He stayed in the cell for almost an hour. 'Don't get too het up. God is looking after you.' Yes, he raised my spirits. In other circumstances I would have found this a ridiculous state of affairs, but there are times when you lose your bearings completely. His words meant more than they would have done elsewhere. And so I ended up more of a 'believer'.

The governor's deputy was next as she made her rounds of the new boys. She advised me to meet the social worker, but first she found out exactly where I'd come from and promised to call my wife. Which she did.

At seven o'clock, dinner was served. The leftover beans with something different: ham. Stewed fish to finish. All that was left was to get on with my two favourite activities: channel-hopping and sleeping.

I didn't want to leave the cell, not even for a walk. As I saw it, being 'outside' didn't mean being in the yard. When I woke up, turning on the television was a reflex action. They were talking about nothing but Willy Voet on all the channels, French, Flemish, Dutch. I felt like the sorcerer's apprentice. My team had had a good chance of winning the Tour, but now they looked set for disaster and it was all my fault. Before such a monumental event, even a small problem can destroy a cyclist's morale . . . I also watched as Jean-Claude Killy, Jean-Marie Leblanc and Bernard Hinault made solemn speeches to the millions of viewers. But what on earth did they take the public for? Who were Hinault and Leblanc trying to convince by saying that they were in a state of total shock, that doping came from another planet. As if they weren't aware that drug-taking is to top-level sport what batons are to a majorette troupe: you rarely find one without the other. Not to mention the moralising being dished out by a television presenter whom I – and others – had once seen sprawled across a sofa in a night club, dead drunk and pulling on a joint.

I was floored by what they were saying, nor did Bruno Roussel's first words give me much comfort either. 'This whole affair has to be looked into. I wish to talk to the police as soon as possible and I want people to leave my cyclists alone.' Would he just drop me – the man who had said that if anything bad should happen, he wouldn't let my wife and children down? I clung on to the memory of these words, but without believing them too much.

And while all this was going on, the president of the UCI, the Dutchman Hein Verbruggen, was on his holidays in Cuba, where the junior world championships were taking place, and in India . . .

I had an irresistible urge to talk to someone, to get it all off my back. Serge was a godsend. He was one of my three warders and the one with whom I got on the best. During his shift he would come and see me two or three times. We would watch television – the hub of prison life – and talk cycling. Before he went home he would pop in and say goodbye.

On the evening of 12 July, fortunately, all we had to do was watch television. From the middle of the afternoon I'd stopped being the main topic of conversation. No one was talking about anything but the World Cup Final. I have a Belgian passport, but, having lived in France for fifteen years, being married to a French woman and having French children, I feel more French than Belgian. For an hour and a half I trembled, thrilled and forgot everything. Ninety minutes of happiness. A shaft of sunlight in a storm-lashed sky.

At the end of the match a camera paused on Trezeguet's tearful face and I wept with him. For I had known the same intensity, the same release of tension, the same pulsating bodies. While the prison rang to the sound of metal plates on the heating pipes, I saw Luc Leblanc becoming world champion at Agrigento in Sicily in 1994, and Laurent Brochard winning the crown at San Sebastian three years later. My tearful eyes were glued to the screen, unable to tear themselves away from the ecstatic crowd surging down the Champs Elysées. And then I saw the Festina riders dancing in their hotel, singing, 'We are the champions!' It was all too much. I almost collapsed. Fortunately the urge to laugh with joy got the upper hand.

On Monday, all the television news was talking about the French soccer team. There was hardly a word for Tom Steels, the stage winner in Dublin, of Chris Boardman's crash on a patch of oil, or Jan Svorada sprinting to victory in Cork. In other words I'd been forgotten and I wasn't unhappy about that. But the newspapers wouldn't let it drop. The prison governor was being kept busy: the telephone simply wouldn't stop ringing. The journalists just wanted to make sure that I was on his premises.

As for me, I was beginning to settle into the strange routine, a mixture of boredom, petty annoyances and television.

FIVE
CHILDREN OF THE PILL

Now I understand Neil Armstrong. I know why, when he came back down to earth, the first thing he did after kissing his wife was to have a shower – an intoxicating, caressing, warm, never-ending shower. There it was, pointing its little rose at me on the morning of 14 July. That Tuesday, as on every Tuesday at Loos, at nine o'clock on the dot, it was shower time. I'd been told about it the evening before and I had thought of nothing else all night. It was a week, to the day, since I had had a wash in hot water – and I was used to having a shower twice a day. All the muck that had gathered – within and without – was washed away with the soapy water. That shower felt like a fifteen-minute purification rite. While the warm, restoring water nursed my skin, my mind wandered back to a time long before this unfortunate July. To where it had all begun.

I was taken back to my childhood, to my grandmother's house, a good kilometre from my parents' home in Hofstade, near Malines, where my brother and I went for a shower every week. The only sanitation at my parents' house was a toilet, so we went over to my grandmother's on a Saturday to be scrubbed clean for Sunday.

My father was a train driver for the SNCB, the Belgian equivalent of British Rail. My mother stayed at home, where she upholstered chairs at the rate of half a dozen a week for a few francs. Back then, football was the main thing we talked about at home. My father played right-back as a semi-professional for the Malines FC. He was a good defender. His win bonuses helped him to buy a small house in 1951. It was only when his football career came to an end that he got on a bike, as a veteran. I started riding at the age of fifteen with the club in Malines, the Dijlespurters, who had a smart white jersey with the Belgian national colours – black, yellow and red – on the back. The sponsor was Pilsor Lamot, a brewery.

I was not a bad racer. In my best-ever season, I won nine races. I took about twenty in total and back then I was racing against the best Belgian juniors of my generation: Eddy Merckx, Herman Van Springel, Walter Godefroot. Once and once only I beat Van Springel, at Kappelen opden Bos. But we didn't really mix, because already these riders brought with them reputations as champions of the future. Merckx was winning about thirty races a year. He was already 'the' Merckx.

Drug-taking was spoken about only in undertones. It was not until 1962, when I was eighteen and had gone up to the senior ranks, that I took my first pills – amphetamines. At that time I wasn't going badly at all. There was a Sunday race near Brussels, at Evere, the town where my uncle and aunt lived. We rode down there with Gérard, who was a good friend of mine in the club. It was the perfect warm-up, about twenty kilometres to get to the start. My dad followed us on his little scooter.

On the way, Gérard whispered that he had got hold of some little white pills. He wouldn't tell me where they had come from, but he insisted, 'You've got good form at the moment, and you're racing with all the family watching. Try them out.' I wasn't keen, but let myself be talked into it. Taking them was so simple. One pill half an hour before the start, the other halfway through the race.

I went up to the registration table after I'd taken the first pill. The hairs on my arms were standing up like porcupine quills and shivers were running up and down my body. The magic potion was working already. I was having to breathe deeply. The second the flag dropped I was off like a bullet from a gun. And I wasn't the only one. I was motoring – I was riding so fast that it scared me. I didn't feel hungry, but on the other hand I had a raging thirst throughout the whole race, which was a loop of about 120 kilometres. And I began to think I was a star! Fuelled by drugs I was able to keep up with guys who were physically stronger and better than me – Willy In'T Ven, Julien Stevens, Georges Pintens, Willy Vekemans, guys who were older than me and on the verge of professional careers; some were to become Merckx's team mates. All big names. And me, the novice – I was the one telling them to get off their backsides and ride. As soon as they saw my face, they caught on. I must have had that look about me . . .

I was spitting fire for about fifteen kilometres. There were six of us in the breakaway, and I felt so strong that I didn't eat anything to keep my strength up. I didn't dare take the second pill: I thought I would burst if I did. The high lasted until about two laps from the finish. And then, all of a sudden, it was as if I had been knocked out. I hit the wall – I couldn't see or hear anything. If someone had walked into the road, I'd have ridden straight into them. I was left behind by the lead group, but somehow managed to hold on to sixth place. In the changing rooms, Gérard passed me the soap. 'Why didn't you eat anything during the race? And why didn't you take the other pill?' Of course, this first try-out hadn't turned me into a winner, but I had felt as strong as an ox, and amphetamines keep calling you back for one more go. Curiosity was replaced by desire.

I remained an amateur until I was twenty-three. As time

went on, my father grew more and more pushy. He liked the atmosphere at races, the smart cars, the chance to rub shoulders with the stars. He wanted me to be one of them. And I was still taking the amphetamines – not at every race, but pretty often, maybe at one race in five, whenever I worked out that I could get a placing.

Starting in my second year as a senior, I'd been going to a masseur, a former professional; it was he who initiated me into another, more pernicious, form of doping. It consisted, not of a pill swallowed at the start, but of a dose taken beforehand over a period of about a week: two solutions of testosterone, which you mixed with water and drank. The effects lasted for two months. It wasn't a little sweetie that you swallowed on impulse; it was premeditated. In short, I dithered, but my father saw where it might lead. I don't know how far he would have gone to make me something that I wasn't – further than I would, anyway.

I left school at eighteen and immediately got a job as a petrol-pump attendant at a garage in Malines, where I stayed for two years. Then, of course, there was no escaping it: fifteen months' national service at Siegen, in Germany, as a colonel's driver. When I got back, my father sent me to a training camp in Italy, organised by a former pro, Desire De Sloove, who owned a big cycle shop in Malines. Two weeks in Desenzano, near Lake Garda, for 6,000 francs. I went with a friend, Johnny Van Camp, and we found ourselves in a little hotel along with several professionals from the Solo Superior team, Van Looy's outfit.

There were four of us to a room: Johnny and I were sharing with a couple of others. On our training rides, when we sometimes did as much as 150 kilometres, the two of us felt absolutely pathetic and came home in a terrible state. The others were as fresh as daisies. In fact, they were powered by amphetamines. One morning, in the toilets, I surprised one of them in the act of injecting something into his arm and the penny dropped. During the two-week training camp, I had lost eight kilos. And in the first few races when I got back to Belgium, I was completely at sea right from the start, completely wasted.

To keep my training going, my father had found me a job as a paper boy. Every morning, at five o'clock, I loaded two hundred newspapers on to my front rack. My butcher's bike alone must have weighed twenty-five kilos, without adding another fifty kilos of papers . . . The round took me the whole morning. That meant that in the afternoon, after a good long siesta, I could go out training – without those damned papers.

After two years, the end of the newspaper round coincided with the death of my small-time career as an amateur. I just couldn't go on any more. My father didn't speak to me for six months. I got a job as a bus driver, on the Malines–Vilvoorde–Brussels line, covering the journey four times a day. I had definitively written off bike racing. And my father had written me off too.

I can't help believing that your fate will always catch up with you some day or other . . . I had just dropped some passengers at a bus stop and as I pulled away I tooted the horn. The guys thought I was hooting at them. They were Ward Janssens and Jef de Schoenmaker, both of whom were racing as professionals. They were lords in the little local kingdom of bike racing. Jef was the son of our butcher and I had raced for years with both of them.

'So you aren't missing the bike, then? Fancy coming to the Grand Prix de Fourmies with us on Sunday?'

Why not? I had nothing in particular to do that weekend. I met Ward Janssens at his house that morning in 1972, some six years after I'd given up on bike racing.

Hanging out with Ward as he travelled around, I got to know Jean de Gribaldy, 'Le Vicomte' (the Viscount). Back then he was team manager of Ward's squad, Magniflex, which he ran with Guillaume Driessens. As the weekends passed, I began to mix with the team personnel. Sometimes Ward asked me to give his legs a massage and he quickly realised that I had good hands.

At the end of 1976, I enrolled at the BLOSO, a well-known sports institute in Ghent, for an eighteen-month course. The programme included lessons in anatomy, first aid and, of course, massage. But I didn't immediately become a wizard like Gus Naessens, Maurice Depauw, Guillaume Michiels or Jeff D'Hondt, who at that time were the demi-gods in the world of the *soigneurs*. They were the ones who could make riders fly. Having your legs in their hands was simultaneously a measure of success and celebrity. It took me eight years to learn the trade and be recognised as a good *soigneur*. To achieve that, you had to have looked after a real champion. But until then I worked at piece rates for one team or another. On any one Sunday I could be hired by Frimatic, the team De Gribaldy was running then, or Safir, Reno, or C&A. I was paid cash, under the counter. Seventy francs a day, a pittance.

I had to wait until 1979 before I actually had a contract in my hand, with Flandria-Ça-va-seul. It was a ten-month contract, of course, ending when the season finished. In the late 1970s only amphetamines could be picked up by the dope controls, which had been brought in after Tom Simpson died on the slopes of Mont Ventoux during the 1967 Tour. But anabolic agents, steroids and corticoids were common currency. And not just amongst some members of the Flandria team.

Of course, the riders didn't really trust me to start with. They looked askance at the new hired hand. It took at least two years to gain their confidence, but I won my spurs courtesy of one of the other *soigneurs*. I watched in his room as he took all the gear out of his huge suitcase, putting it on a table as if dressing a shop window. Pirate treasure.

He was the one who taught me my profession, showing me many things but concealing many more. I was tolerated back then: admission to this parallel universe was not automatic. When a rider came to his room to ask for a sleeping pill, he would turn the key in the lock. The mystique had to be maintained even if there was nothing to hide – to a ridiculous degree, on occasion. One day another *soigneur* made a colossal cock-up. As part of the climate of secrecy, all the labels on the bottles were switched – he would even swap his massage creams around. The problem arose when this guy had to put grease on the chamois leather insert in Walter Planckaert's shorts and mixed up the jars. Instead of using cold cream, which would stop the shorts rubbing on his crutch, he slapped on hot oil meant for the legs! Walter can probably remember it to this day . . .

My apprenticeship was largely based on experience. You had to keep your eyes and ears open, gleaning sketchy information from gestures, snatches of conversation and phrases here and there, and patiently putting it all back together. It was essential to talk things over with the riders because they knew everything. It defies belief that even today, after a positive drug test, they will swear on the grave of their mother that they were given drugs without their knowledge. They have always known exactly what they are taking. Probably better than I used to: because they know their own bodies, how they react, what moment to put something in, what drug to take, and what dose. Riding as a professional means being professional on every level. But, as they tend to say with a big smile, 'I've never taken anything, it's always been given to me.' In actual fact, only Belgian mix is a real mystery, even for the cyclists, because the ingredients vary from mix to mix. It's real junk. It may be heavy stuff, but it's the poor man's amphetamine. In 1980 its ancestors were called Tonedron and Pervitin, the legendary 'Tonton' and 'Tintin', but by comparison these were 'clean' substances.

In short, when the cogs are well oiled, the *soigneur* is basically carrying out orders, limiting himself to measuring out carefully calculated doses and mixing up potions. But it takes a long time for a *soigneur*–rider team to fulfil its potential. It's no coincidence that the best *soigneurs* look after the best riders. In 1979 I had three or four in my care, including Joaquim Agostinho who finished third in the Tour de France. To start with, all I did was massage them. I didn't take care of them in every sense, it was a gradual process of evolution. My first intravenous injection, which was stuff to help recovery, was on Janssens. 'You'd better get your hand in,' he said. I was white with nerves.

'Bang it in, go on, bang it in! Look, that vein's like a motorway!'

I was trembling like a leaf. So he took me by the hand and guided the syringe home. It went in like a knife through butter.

So then I went through the full spectrum. Amphetamines injected into the arm or the stomach, corticoids, steroids, anabolic agents, even testosterone injected into the buttock muscles. Daily rituals, nothing out of the ordinary. No one thought of it as fraud, cheating or dangerous. Only amphetamines were forbidden in theory because they were liable to show up in urine tests. But until the start of the 1980s drug tests were as sophisticated as a gasworks . . .

For important races, or to build up to events that had been specifically targeted, a capsule of Decca-Dorabulin 25 or 50 was injected on top of the usual mix. It's a male hormone, an anabolic. The riders who took it knew themselves by heart and would drop a Decca–Dorabulin 25 a week before the start of the Tour and another about halfway through the race, before the start of the mountain stages. The upside: they would feel the effects for a month. The downside: the stuff was detectable in the urine for a long time.

For the one-day Classics, depending on what their racing programme was, many would take an ampoule of Synacten Delayed or Immediate, which stimulates the adrenal glands, making them produce cortisone. As the period of the opening Classics lasts for six weeks, from mid-March to the end of April, they would gradually step up their intake every three days.

And they often turned to amphetamines as well. There were drug tests only in the biggest races: the Tours of France, Spain and Italy, the one-week stage races, the one-day Classics and semi-Classics. For the rest, in the Chargers' Grand Prix – the mocking nickname given to races where anything went – the riders charged up with impunity.

But all this wasn't going to come to an end because of one big scandal in the Tour de France. Quite the contrary . . .

SIX
TUBE UP THE BUM

No one had warned me. Not even Serge, who was obviously having a day off. It was a complete surprise, almost a shock. That Friday, 17 July, in other words on the seventh day that I was shut up in Loos, a warder opened the cell door.

'Visiting room.'

Visiting room? I may have lived in France for fifteen years, but there are words and situations that I have trouble working out immediately. Visiting room . . . In the corridor I worked out that someone had come to see me, but I assumed it was my lawyer, Ludovic Baron. Before entering the visiting room I had to be searched, as the rules stated, then we went through several doors and past several warders before plunging into a long corridor with numbered glass openings.

'Gate 16.'

Going in, I saw her, sitting there with a little smile on her lips. It was my Sylvie. My God, the sight of her made me happy.

We just sat there looking at each other, crying. There was a table between us, and under the table transparent plastic, but we could touch each other. Talking was a different matter, though. I had spent so much time imagining how it would be when we met again and now we were struck dumb with emotion.

Eventually the words came and we talked about everything under the sun: Charlotte and Mathieu, our children, who were being looked after by Eric Caritoux, a bike rider who lived nearby; the Lille police searching our house; the lawyer who was going to defend me, Jean-Louis Bessis, who had been recommended to my wife because of a difficult case which he had won against the extreme right a few years earlier, and who was going to be important, given the proportions of the affair; the house, the phone calls, all the fall-out from the meteorite which had fallen on our heads.

As this was her first visit, Sylvie was permitted two visiting periods back to back, a full hour and a half. She told me that Bruno Roussel had phoned her from Ireland, that he had said the Festina team would look after everything, including my family, if I ended up in prison for a long spell. But I had to state that the stuff which I was carrying around was intended for my personal consumption. This demand had merely made my wife more worried, as all she knew about what had happened to me came from the television news. And she had grown more concerned when Bruno told her to burn my notebooks. She had kept them safe.

We said goodbye a dozen times when we heard the footsteps of the warder in the corridor and a dozen times we joined hands to comfort each other. When I got back to the cell it occurred to me that the earthquake was only just beginning and another scandal came to mind.

The scandal, the great scandal, gave everyone pause for thought. And it had been bound to happen one day. On 16 July 1978, on the mountain top at l'Alpe d'Huez, the Belgian Michel Pollentier, riding for the Flandria team, had just taken the Tour de France's yellow jersey from Joseph Bruyère, after winning the stage from Hennie Kuiper and Bernard Hinault.

Proud as a peacock, Pollentier headed for the caravan where the drug test was taking place without any fears. Routine stuff, but everyone knows the story now. He had a rubber bulb under his arm, with a tube attached to the bulb running down through his long-sleeved jersey as far as his wrist, where it was stopped with a little cork. It should have been easy. All Pollentier had to do was deliver a small quantity of urine that wasn't his. But the whole set-up had been sabotaged, which is something the media have never reported, for the simple reason that they didn't know. The pipe was blocked. Pollentier began to get het up, he started sweating, and the doctor who was running the test got suspicious when the Belgian refused point-blank to get undressed to cool down. The Tour collapsed into farce.

Disqualified, thrown off the race, Pollentier was banned for two months. But, more seriously, in the eyes of the world the sport of cycling had been caught red-handed.

It was Fred De Bruyne, who was Pollentier's team manager at the time, who told me the story behind the story one day when we were going through the myriad ways of evading drug tests. And he warned me: 'Don't gamble too much on it, because when it all flies up and hits you in the face it's very painful.'

Since then no one, as far as I know, has risked using this system again, but human nature is ingenious and men never give up. This, presumably, is what leads to progress. Examples of human ingenuity are legion – they include the 'hidey hole', which I learned somewhere along the way from a Belgian *soigneur* with the Ijsboerke team.

You have to get a rubber tube, which is both flexible and rigid. At one end you fix a small cork, at the other a condom, running about a third of the way up the tube. Finally, just as a precaution, you stick carpet pile, or any short hair, on the part of the tube which isn't in the condom.

In the team car, when the rider comes to change before going to the drug control, you go on to stage two: you slip the part of the tube fitted with the condom up the backside, inject clean urine up the tube with a large syringe, cork it and stick it to the skin, following the line of the perineum, as far as the testicles. That's why the hairs are necessary, to hide the tube in case the doctor running the test decides to lean down. The condom full of urine is held in the anus, which has the advantage of keeping the urine at body temperature, so the doctor won't be suspicious, as he would be if presented with a flask of cold liquid. This system was never bettered – no doctor suspected a thing and I used it for three years without any worries.

I tried it out for the first time on a little-known rider from the Marc Zeep Central team. It went like clockwork. The device was reliable, quick to set up and soon being used by the riders. A great one-day Classic specialist saw for himself how well it worked after he won the Tour of Flanders. However, it was not for the faint-hearted. You can't be too squeamish if you're going to walk towards the doctor in charge of the dope test with something like that up your backside. Cyclists are warriors on the bike, but they are good actors off it. Since Pollentier's catastrophe, in principle the riders were meant to take their clothes off for the test. Nothing could be hidden under their arms or in their pockets. So another hiding place had to be found . . .

In spite of the small number of cyclists let into the secret – mainly Belgians – the word gradually spread. I found out that the system had died a death a few years later. As usual, in his delight at fiddling a dope control, a rider or a *soigneur* had spoken about it in confidence to one of his colleagues, who did the same thing, and so on until a well-known German cyclist was caught at a control on home turf. It had all been a secret, of course.

★ ★ ★

To get round the powers of the dope control, there were simpler methods. Far simpler. According to the doctor, and the mood he was in, it was often possible for a cyclist to remain in his shorts while he urinated into the sample jar in a compartment with the door open. If the cyclist had managed to slip a flask of clean urine into the leg of his shorts, that was that. All I had to do was to distract the doctor's attention at the critical moment. And there were many more tricks.

On the other hand, if the rider was forced to undress completely, it was somewhat harder on the nerves, but we never lost our cool. While my 'client' began to get worried, to drink on the pretext that he was having trouble passing water because of dehydration, I would pick up his shorts with the flask inside. It might be a long wait, but at some point I would always find a way to place the little container in a corner of the caravan, behind the curtain, at the back of the cistern in the toilet, anywhere. As soon as the doctor lost patience and got up or went somewhere, the rider would discreetly pick up the flask. The medic would always crack before we did. After all, no matter how scrupulous they were, they were only doctors, not customs men.

There were so many other ways and means, like the bandage on the arm, which could be used to store clean urine. Very convenient for a stage race. We would tell the press that such and such a rider had been injured but, riding on pure courage alone, he would be starting the stage that day. There would be no question about the bandage and it would all seem completely natural. When we were putting on the plaster, we would slide in a metal container; it would be taken out and in the space where it had been we would insert a condom full of clean urine.

The instinct to cheat would lead some riders to the most painful remedies imaginable. In some teams the doctor, who might happen to be a specialist in urology, would extract the riders' urine before they took the drugs. Just in case. If need be, he would put a syringe about two centimetres up their urethra to inject the clean urine before they went to the control after the race. They just had to grin and bear it. And they did.

At the start of the 1980s, I invented another way round the controls, which was christened 'double sides' and was used as a last resort. All you needed was a flask on which a band of 'double-sided' tape was stuck – the same stuff you use at home for sticking down carpet. I would only take the plastic strip off the other side at the last minute, just before 'going to work' to avoid any dust gathering. In the drug-test caravan, the cyclist would go towards the toilet and pass in front of me – at the point where he couldn't be seen I would gently stick the flask on his back. He would then go into the toilet and swap over the urine. You just need to use your imagination.

Unfortunately, there were circumstances which couldn't be foreseen, such as the way some riders sweat at the finish of a race. One day the 'double side' slipped off and the flask fell to the floor. Fortunately, the doctor had his back turned. I immediately covered up the evidence with the rider's jersey and my rucksack, yelling out, 'Oh, shit,' as if I had just dropped them. We had got away with it again.

You couldn't avoid some farcical scenes. The finest I saw was not down to a cyclist but to his wife, at a drug test at l'Alpe d'Huez, at the finish of a Tour de France stage in 1979. It was very embarrassing for the rider in question. He was not brilliant in the mountains, so that morning he had slipped himself an amphetamine 'pick-me-up'. Not to outdo the proper climbers, merely to finish within the time limit for the stage. But I had warned him, 'Watch out, you know. This isn't a village fête, it's the Tour. You might be picked out for the random test.' He said heartily, 'That's about as likely as a pigeon crapping on my head as I leave the hotel.'

When he got to the dope-control caravan, where the names of the chosen few had been posted an hour before the finish, he realised that the pigeon had been on target after all . . .

So it was time for a salvage operation. There was only one thing to do in an emergency like this: slip the flask into his shorts. Then it was down to him to look after himself. But there was no way this doctor was going to be distracted for a single second. He was particularly tenacious. The look of the cyclist, a former champion who had been brought low by imbibing too much magic potion, spoke volumes. There was nothing he could do. I was as annoyed as he was . . .

I was sweating so hard that I had to leave the caravan. Outside I bumped into his wife, who was making a flying visit to the Tour.

'Is he going to be in there for long, Willy?'

I explained to her that the situation was becoming critical. To my huge surprise, she didn't give a damn.

'That'll teach him!'

I was still trying to figure a way out when, all of a sudden, just behind me, she collapsed in a faint.

'Doctor, doctor! A woman has just been taken ill!'

The policeman who was keeping an eye on the area around the dope-control area began beating on the door of the caravan. Only thinking of his duty to the sick, the doctor burst out to see to the stricken woman. Two or three pats on the back later she regained consciousness. That was far more time than her husband needed once he had been left on his own.

'It's nothing. Just the heat, I reckon.'

The cyclist didn't boast about this one when he got back to the team hotel.

To understand how things are in dope-control caravans,

you only have to listen to the words which the riders exchange as they go in and out. Just like schoolboys coming out of an exam, they swap fleeting words, and make sympathetic faces, things like, 'It's OK, the doctor's cool,' and, 'Watch out, he looks at everything,' or, 'You have to take them all off.' This is why it was always best not to go in first, so you could make a plan of action.

The thing which worked above all else when going to the dope control was to be one of the greats. Like borrowing from a bank which only lends money to the rich, and which gives flowers to its best customers, a famous cyclist had a lot more chance of dodging the system. That's how it is, the effects of celebrity extend to the edge of a toilet seat in a dope-control caravan. Even the doctors would be impressed at the thought of being with one of the stars, if only for a few minutes: time for an autograph, a handshake, a kind word, a smile. A star could be caught red-handed and not have to pay the price.

All this subterfuge came to an end in the mid-1980s. More and more often the winner of a race would go straight from the presentation podium to the dope control. There was no chance to go via the team bus to 'get changed'. The strengthening of the drug tests, which became more methodical, made it harder to play at hide-and-seek. And amphetamines were used less and less in races, apart from at the start of the season. The drug tests only began in March, at Paris–Nice and Milan–San Remo, not before. But out training no one had any inhibitions. Spot checks only began a lot later. The usual method back then was to cut in half the tube of a syringe containing a small amount of amphetamine and stick it – or sew it – to the inside of the jersey, level with the stomach. At the right moment, in the needle went.

As for the undetectable drugs, they were still in their

heyday. Cortisone was undetectable in the urine, and that's still the case; testosterone would be flushed out of the system four days after it was taken, and some anabolic agents would disappear after a week . . . So the chargers can still say as they always have: no positive tests, no doping. And they have ended up being convinced of it. It's as though you made the following equation: 180 kilometres per hour on the motorway with no speed camera means you're inside the speed limit.

SEVEN

FANCY A FRUIT BAR WITH EYES?

The judge had promised that I wouldn't be kept inside for more than a week. It was now 20 July 1998 and I'd been moping in my cell for ten days. Two days earlier the whole Festina team had been thrown off the Tour, a piece of news that I couldn't come to terms with. Seen over again and again, the pictures of a weeping Virenque coming out of the café Chez Guillou in Corrèze after holding his last press conference pierced my heart, made me feel like a thief who had seen the light. Because of me, the high hopes of the best cycling team in the world had been reduced to dust. I wallowed in my grief in the same way that my serving of vegetables washed around the tin plate. The idea of getting out of the slammer gave me goosebumps. I imagined a lynch mob waiting for me at the gate to punish me for unleashing this whirlwind. Without realising it, I'd pressed the red button and started a war.

I was turning these dark thoughts over and over in my head when the warder came for me.

'Come on. There are two policemen waiting for you.'

It was all about to start again. What were they going to do with me this time? What with body searches, threats and interrogations, I didn't know where I was any more.

They introduced themselves, before telling me what they had come for. I had to provide proof that I really did work for the Festina team, as I said I did. Of course, I had no identification on me, so they took me back to the office where I'd handed in my things. They recovered my briefcase and rucksack, which had surely been gone through already with a fine-tooth comb. It didn't matter; they began rummaging through my things again: my underwear, the fax inviting me to the Tour, my credit cards. And in the end they kept the one thing they had come to find: my 'road book' for the current season. This personal organiser, to which no one had paid any attention so far, now became an incriminating item. The two cops were quite nice about it and we had a friendly chat, without any undercurrents of tension. One of them was even so good as to explain that 'importing substances dangerous to health' might be going to cost me dear.

'Why don't you ask to be seen by the judge before you are summoned on Friday? Just a matter of getting things out into the open. We'll see to it for you if you want.'

I could only agree, the more so because I'd prevaricated the first time I'd been before the judge. I had explained to him that the stuff was brought in in the team's equipment lorry, but he clearly hadn't believed me: this time, on 23 July, he asked me for the name of the person who had brought the stuff into France. I was caught. I stuttered a bit, then suggested he ask the same question on the following day, when Roussel, Rijckaert and I were to be questioned together in the same room – the 'confrontation'. 'I would prefer Bruno Roussel to answer that question. If he won't say, I will tell you.' The judge acquiesced.

Fortunately, Bruno Roussel saved me the trouble. In the end he was one of the few people, perhaps the only person at a management level, to accept responsibility for his actions and to realise that lying gets you nowhere. Ultimately, it's all self-deception.

FANCY A FRUIT BAR WITH EYES?

During my first years as a full-time *soigneur*, with the Belgian teams Flandria, Marc Zeep Centrale and Daf-Trucks, from 1979 to 1981, I found out that for the majority of riders cheating could become a way of life. It just depended on the situation. I can remember the Tour of Germany in the spring of 1979, the year it came back on the international calendar after not being run for several years.

Before the race finish in Dortmund, where everyone expected the great German rider Dietrich Thurau to take overall victory, there was one really hard stage, with a hill six miles long just after the start. One of the Flandria riders, Albert Van Vlierberghe, a decent Belgian racer but with no taste for the hills, decided that he wasn't going up it.

'Take me in the car. The guys will set off flat out, I know what they're like, and I'll be chasing my backside off all day.'

I was still new to the job and didn't really dare to say no to one of the cyclists. But I was nervous, on his account as well as mine.

'Don't worry, Willy. If anyone catches sight of me we can say that I pulled out, it's easy enough.'

And so we set off in the car a quarter of an hour before the start, him with a *soigneur*'s jacket on his shoulders and me with butterflies in my stomach. We got to the top, where the road flattened out, and parked by a barn at the roadside. I left him there – I had to see to the *bidons* for the riders – hidden behind the barn, waiting for the best moment to catch up with the race as if nothing had happened. Everything panned out exactly as he had expected: the bunch had split to pieces as soon as the flag had been dropped, and this made it easy for him. After the first race vehicles had passed through – mainly press cars – he slipped into no man's land between the breakaway of about ten riders and the front of the bunch. He caught up with the lead group without any problems, and – best of all – he was able to finish sixth on the stage.

There are many examples like this. Brute strength is often worth nothing compared to a little brain power. And brain power can be used in many ways, as I saw on the Tour of Flanders once around the same time. The 'Ronde' was really something, especially for Flandrians like me – a hard man's race over 250 kilometres of little hills, some cobbled. The course is so compact that by cutting across it and back again spectators can see the race go past several times.

On the quiet little road leading into the finish I remember meeting a good rider who wasn't one of my team. Clearly, to judge by the speed he was going, he had pulled out of the race. I asked him if he wanted me to take him to the finish in the car and he signed his thanks with one hand.

'No, no. I'll ride down there, thanks all the same. It'll just be a few more miles in my legs for the day.'

I left him to his training ride and went on my way again. An hour before the finish, I was talking to the other *soigneurs* on the finish line when the loudspeakers spat out a name – the name of the rider I had met a few hours before!

He obviously hadn't planned it that way. He had got mixed up with the race and had latched on as they went past. This might have been the case, but I still had my doubts – his brother raced as a professional as well. I thought they might have been mixed up.

At the finish it was the usual scrum and I forgot about this perplexing issue until I got to the dope control. Who was down on the list of riders who had to deliver a sample, having finished second? 'My' impostor, who had covered eighty kilometres less that day than the rest of the opposition. Out of sight, out of mind, as always.

We bumped into each other again a few weeks later. When I recalled his superb exploit and took the mickey, he pretended not to understand at first. Then, as I looked at him with a mixture of amusement and disbelief, he ended the conversation: 'Just keep your mouth shut, anyway.'

These tricks are as nothing compared to what can be achieved when a doctor and a rider work in tandem. One particular Liège–Bastogne–Liège at the end of the 1970s speaks volumes. 'Liège' is one of cycling's monuments, the oldest of the one-day Classics on one of the toughest courses; it is also one of the most sought after because it can be won only by a real all-rounder at the peak of his form.

The rider in question had prepared himself accordingly, using 'all available technology'. He had no fears because the doctor who was in charge of the drug testing was his own doctor! A doctor who oversaw the preparation of several top cyclists while also doing anti-doping work for the Federation. Another Rijckaert, in other words, because Eric worked for the Flemish authorities as well. These doctors were appointed by the Ministry of Sport to take care of drug testing, not only at bike races, but also at football matches and boxing tournaments. These Rijckaerts could be found everywhere – in Italy, in France – with a whole crowd of cyclists as 'patients' . . . And it's still the same today.

It's worth pointing out that most of the doctors who 'prepared' cyclists did not leave a trail of carnage in their wake. A doctor like Rijckaert would try to manage the ever-growing demands made on him by his clients. I remember as well that he refused to sign the licence of a Belgian rider in whom he had diagnosed a cardiac anomaly when he examined him at the start of the season. The kid went elsewhere. Nine months later he died of a heart attack on the bike.

In the 1980s everything was worth trying. A senior one-day specialist came to beef up the team where I was working. He arrived with a fine racing record and a well-stocked briefcase. Being kindly disposed towards me, he didn't hide anything about his medical preparation. He told me about the banned drugs he used, but also about the right way to use them and about his recuperation techniques. This guy really took me a long way up the ladder because it's not enough merely to know what drugs to use – you have to inject them at the right moment and know how to calculate the proportions if you're mixing them. The older *soigneurs* had not told me everything, but I don't hold it against them. That's how I've always behaved with new *soigneurs*. It's up to them to find out for themselves, just as I did.

One day, just after the Tour de France, this rider announced that he was going to win a big race in a few weeks. During the ten days before the race he put himself on a course of Synacten Retard – delayed-action cortisone – an injection every two days. The day of the race, half an hour before the start, he took an injection of Synacten Immediate – a drug still used widely today for the major one-day Classics because it is undetectable. He knew exactly what he needed at any given moment and the result was never in doubt.

But it didn't always work out that well. I remember a Tour of Lombardy in the 1980s. The morning of the start, the rider who went on to win the race eight hours later took an injection of Synacten Immediate in his backside, into the muscle, so that the effects would be felt gradually. At the first feeding zone, the field was all over the place, and he was two minutes behind a break that had formed early on. But although he had not started off well, at the second feed, two-thirds of the way through the race, he caught the leading riders. Then he came good and won on his own. Initially, the cold and the overdose of cortisone had produced the opposite result from the one expected and actually slowed him down. The rider hadn't been put off and had dug deep to go into overdrive towards the end. Being the strong man he was, he might well have won without any outside assistance. But just as money doesn't create happiness but goes a long way towards it, doping doesn't create a champion but doesn't do him any harm either.

Another case where a rider miscalculated was the so-called 'feat' achieved by Bert Oosterbosch, a superb Dutch time triallist, in the Grand Prix des Nations in 1982. The race consisted of two laps of a forty-five kilometre circuit around Cannes. At the first time check, after eighteen kilometres, Oosterbosch, who specialised in short events, was eighteenth, one and a half minutes behind the leader. Halfway through he was eleventh; after seventy-five kilometres the Dutch redhead was fourth, just under three minutes behind the eventual winner, Bernard Hinault, and in the end he took third, less than two and a half minutes behind 'the Badger'. He finished like a thunderbolt, and the press sang his praises for the way in which he had calculated his efforts, especially on the long ascent to Vallauris.

There was a completely different explanation, however. The Synacten Immediate which he had taken shortly before the start had actually made him go more slowly, but even though he needed both feet to get one pedal to move, he didn't panic. Instead of giving up, he waited patiently for his system to clear up. The Synacten just kicked in an hour late, but it was one hour too late for him to win the race.

In any list of the subterfuges we used to conceal the drugs, it's impossible to leave out 'fruit bars with eyes'. Even when it was still possible to race on amphetamines – and there are still Chargers' Grands Prix, even today – it didn't seem like a good idea to let everyone see them. So we went through this charade to conceal the little pills, five milligrammes of Pervitin or Captagon: we stuck them in a fruit bar. We would stick them in like eyes, with a nose on top if the rider wanted three. I've known guys take up to 100 milligrammes in a race, in which case we stuck on not a face but a whole skeleton! In the morning, in the hotel, when I went from room to room asking who wanted eyes, a nose, even a mouth, in his fruit bar, everyone understood. Doping, in any shape or form, has always been an integral part of the culture of top-level cycling.

There was one case at least where the whole panoply of drugs, Immediate, Retard, 200 milligrammes, 500 milligrammes, quick-acting or slow-burn, was rendered totally useless. It was at the world championship at Goodwood, in England, in 1982, where I was working with the Belgian team. The night before the race, Freddy Maertens, one of the biggest stars of the team, rolled up at the hotel in a taxi. There was no sign of life for a moment, but just as we got worried, lo and behold, there he was walking through the restaurant towards us, pissed as a newt. He might be the defending world champion, but it hadn't stopped him getting totally plastered. Given how drunk he was, there wasn't a lot we could do. We thought about giving him a pick-up, but he was already off in a deep sleep. Next morning, he completed three laps of the circuit and made a speedy exit.

The links between a rider and *soigneur* aren't necessarily based on putting their heads together to formulate the perfect preparation for D-Day, as is shown by what happened during another Tour of Lombardy in the 1980s.

The evening before this Italian Classic, we had driven to the team presentation in two cars. As our team manager still had to go to the managers' meeting, the rest of us squeezed into an estate car to drive back to the hotel. This particular rider took the wheel and I ended up in the boot among the riders' bags.

He was never slow when it came to winding people up. To amuse the other riders, he began swerving all over the place and slamming on the brakes. I was being thrown from side to side in the back. The more I yelled, the more wildly he drove, until I ended up smashing my head on the car roof.

Back at the hotel, I didn't waste time telling him what I thought: 'God, you wind me up. Just because you're a star doesn't mean you can just do anything you like!'

We had a lengthy shouting match. That evening I didn't say a word to him while I was massaging his legs. And when the time came to minister to his other needs, notably the cortisone injection, I got a bottle ready with a very bad grace and threw it down on the bedside table.

'There's your shit. Good night.'

He had to fend for himself, which didn't seem to trouble him in the slightest. The next morning we still weren't friends: we cut each other dead.

A few hours later he crossed the line with his arms in the air. I was in the area behind the finish and he saw me as he slowed down. We fell into each other's arms and cried like a pair of kids.

The variety of drugs on offer is so large that there is stuff to suit all tastes. Although cycling is an endurance sport, riders also take stimulants, some of which are authorised by sports federations although they are damaging to the body. This is the case with caffeine injected into the muscle, which is useful in time trials and mountain stages, but above all with Trinitrin. This drug contains a huge dose of caffeine and acts immediately on the heart. The sprinters know all about it: five or six kilometres before the final sort-out the chargers pop a pill and the effect is almost immediate. It's the same in prologue time trials, which are about brief, violent effort. As far as I know, riders stopped using this at the start of the 1990s, because, although it was tolerated, it was still dangerous if used regularly.

And I would say that about 60 per cent of the pack was

in the grip of drugs. Not always the same people, or the same drugs, mind. There was a constant rotation between the riders who, for example, were coming back after an injury, those who had objectives later in the year and were merely building up their strength, those who were at the end of a racing programme and about to take a rest, and the ones who wanted to win on a particular day. And some were capable of taking on a bigger workload than others, finishing three major Tours a year without buckling under the strain. That is the way of nature.

Another widely used procedure was suppositories into which caffeine – or sometimes amphetamines – had been injected. We would get pharmacists to make up suppositories of 200 or 300 milligrammes. There were even riders who asked for suppositories of 500 milligrammes, which was over the legal limit. The pharmacists, who weren't stupid, knew what they were used for, but shut their eyes. The suppositories were wrapped up in aluminium foil, so that they wouldn't melt, and put in a Thermos bottle, which I kept with me. When we got to the feeding station where I was to hand up the riders' food bags, I would stick them to the *bidons* with sellotape and slip them into the food bags. These were known as 'parachute *bidons*'. With eighty kilometres left to the finish, to get ready for the final key phase of the race, all the riders had to do was get on the plane . . .

At the start of every season, I would order from a Belgian pharmacy 2,000 small, transparent plastic tubes to use at the start of a race. I would place inside them the following items: at the bottom of the tube, a dark brown pill, Anémine, which is caffeine, taking care not to exceed 400 milligrammes, then a yellow one, Hexacine, or Coltramyl, which was white, to combat cramp and finally a green one, Thiocticide, to reduce the production of toxins. These were covered with a bit of cotton wool, on which I placed another three pills: red, Persentin, a pick-me-up which enables the rider to find his second wind quickly; white, Berevine B1, another substance which hinders the effect of toxins on the muscles; and finally transparent yellow, vitamin E, to combat fatigue.

The riders didn't make systematic use of these concoctions, which didn't actually contain anything against the rules. Everything depended on how the race went, on their state of fitness and their place in the race. I had to order so many little tubes because the riders simply threw them away as they took the pills. When I think how many of them must be lying in ditches around Europe . . .

The general public has found out since last year that the system which Bruno Roussel set up was intended partly to prevent riders taking drugs with no understanding of the consequences. But ten years earlier they acted on their own initiative as much as they do now, and it was just as dangerous. The riders were left to their own curiosity and the greed of people who did not have their interests at heart. Some things never change.

EIGHT

MADMAN'S MIX

He visited me every afternoon, except at the weekend. On Tuesday 21 July he didn't diverge from this habit. I met him at the *etoile*, a meeting place on the ground floor, and we shut ourselves into an office which was specifically for this kind of meeting. My lawyer, Ludovic Baron, was a good guy. We spoke to each other using the informal *tu* because it comes easily to me. Back in Belgium everyone is called *tu*, apart from your priest, your doctor and your banker. And that's the kind of person I am.

He told me at once that the 'confrontation' between Bruno Roussel, Eric Rijckaert and myself – where we would be placed face to face and presented with each other's evidence – would take place on 24 July at nine-thirty. I was desperate to meet them again. I knew that both of them had initially denied the evidence and contradicted my statements and I was keen to establish the truth in front of the judge. They had both been placed under formal investigation and were under more suspicion than I was, but I was afraid that greater weight would be attached to the words of an employer and of a doctor who had signed the Hippocratic oath than to the guy who did the fetching and carrying. It would be their word against mine, as we looked each other in the eye. It was a situation in which individuals are made to accept responsibility, with only their conscience as their judge.

There are those who still weep for Le Vicomte, as we used to call Jean de Gribaldy. A character, a man to be reckoned with. Cycling is full of champions, of personalities, and De Gribaldy has a central place in its family photograph. The two years I spent at his side, 1982 and 1983, have marked me for ever.

De Gribaldy was an independent spirit and deeply sensitive, but at the same time he kept a certain distance from the cyclists, addressing them with the formal *vous*. He was hot-blooded and cold at the same time. He was one of the first to recognise the importance of nutrition to a sportsman and would not tolerate any divergence from a strict diet. Back then, the riders were not as thin as rakes like they are now, but tended to be a few pounds overweight. At the start of the season they would charge up with amphetamines, as much to lose weight as to be up there in the races.

Le Vicomte knew of only one method of losing weight: just eat less. Burning as many calories as they do, cyclists are always hungry, but the old man would watch over his flock with total intransigence. I remember the first training camp his Sem-France-Loire team held at Mandelieu on the Côte d'Azur in February 1983. He hid everything – bread, butter, wine. The riders were left to eat dry toast. They were so hungry that instead of hanging around in their rooms before dinner, they were queuing up in the restaurant at seven-thirty. Le Vicomte would even resort to putting bromide in their food so they would eat less, but he would also put yeast extract on their salad or their pasta – an excellent sauce. It's a practice I've maintained. The yeast extract – not the bromide.

The team he ran was high-class: Sean Kelly, Steven Rooks, Jean-Marie Grezet, René Bittinger . . . These last two were in the hands of Pierre Ducrot, a masseur and osteopath whom I had met in 1979, and who later went on to look after Gilles Delion at the Helvetia team. Ducrot had spent all his career with Le Vicomte, and had followed him to Sem-France-Loire. Our approaches were completely different, to say the least, and we had more than a few arguments. He was preaching in the wilderness: he simply didn't want to hear about medicine, let along about drugs, but gave priority to diet and homeopathy. And Jean de Gribaldy had complete faith in him.

Le Vicomte went as far as preparing the *bidons* himself. It may have been the *soigneurs'* job to look after the riders' food, but you never know . . . He would shut himself in his room and let no one in. I learned later that he was suspicious of everyone and was afraid of dodgy stuff being put in the bottles.

It was with Sem-France-Loire that I gained my reputation as a *soigneur*. More precisely, it was with Sean Kelly. A fantastic one-day Classic specialist, with ten to his credit during his career: Paris–Roubaix twice; Milan–San Remo twice, Liège–Bastogne– Liège twice, the Tour of Lombardy three times, as well as Blois–Chaville, not to mention Ghent–Wevelgem, the Grand Prix des Nations, a Tour of Spain and stages in every big race. As a rider he was indifferent to pain, and his career lasted almost twenty years. He was one of a rare breed. Before you can be a champion you have to be made of special stuff.

We met at the end of the 1970s. Back then, he lived in Vilvoorde on the outskirts of Brussels, about five miles from my house, which made it easy to get to know him. Even though he rode for a different team, he often came to my house for a massage, paying me a daily rate. So I got to know him physically and mentally because you must never lose sight of the fact that every rider has to be prepared specifically. Because individuals are unique, you can't stick to any sort of rigid method.

A recent story illustrates the point. In spring 1998 Laurent Dufaux had just won the Tour of Romandie by a street. He was absolutely flying, using cortisone, a fact which didn't escape his team mate and fellow-Swiss Alex Zülle, who had arrived at the team in the off-season. Less than a week before the Tour of Italy, for which he was the favourite, Alex, who was the Festina leader on the race, came and asked for the same course of treatment.

'All you need to power you is your class. It will be more than enough for the prologue.'

Alex was strong enough anyway, the more so because he'd been using a treatment based on growth hormone to prepare him before he moved on to corticosteroids. When you are tuning up a Formula One car, you deal with the tyres, the engine, and the aerodynamics one by one. Every parameter has to be just perfect. It's the same with a cyclist. You can work out after every stage of a race what state the rider is in, depending on his blood-test readings and the graph traced by the heart-rate monitor which he wears during the race. You can foresee breakdown or improvement.

The Spanish *soigneur* who looked after Zülle's preparation just carried on regardless. He thought that he could apply to Alex a method which had worked on another rider. So he injected massive doses of corticosteroids, which destroyed the balance which had been so finely calculated. Where the hormones had been building up the muscle, the 'cortico' just devoured them. The result was disastrous: after being by far the strongest in the first ten days, Alex simply fell to bits.

My divorce from my first wife at the start of the 1984 season was traumatic, so much so that when the Tour of Spain finished in early May, I decided to get a change of air to sort my life out and clear my head. I came back at the start of June, working on a day rate for a small French team.

The squad included a larger-than-life character who was

very attached to the Bordeaux–Paris one-day race. This event doesn't exist any more, and it has to be said that it was symbolic of another era. The start was at eleven o'clock at night in Bordeaux. The riders rode together, warmly dressed, as far as Poitiers, where they arrived early in the morning. There, for about an hour, they would change their clothes and have a bite to eat and a massage, before being sent off behind small motorbikes known as Dernys to race to Paris. That was when the race began in earnest, but the whole event was a fearsome, fascinating show.

That year, the rider in question was on heavy fuel. We had hardly left Poitiers before he rode alongside the car, clearly in a stew.

'Fucking hell, give me my injection now!'

It wasn't safe. There was always the chance that there might be a witness in one of the cars, which would be embarrassing. It just wasn't the right time to pull his shorts down, sterilise the skin with a bit of cotton and surgical spirit, bung the needle in through the window, rub the buttock to spread the dope around and pull the shorts back up.

'I don't give a toss. Just get the damn' syringe in me. Get on with it!'

I did it with the syringe through the shorts. He put his arms around my neck in Paris and sighed. 'God, Willy, did I feel good or what? Bloody good job you stopped me on the finish line or I'd be in Lille by now!'

Bordeaux–Paris was a race that was too inhuman for a rider to get through without some help. I knew one winner, a Belgian, who wasn't particularly into drugs but demanded a special prescription for this particular event. An injection of Kenacort in one buttock to get him through the first six hours, then hydrocortisone pills to get him to the finish. He would head for home with a light heart and a clear conscience. The drug test would never pick up a thing. It was a demanding race for the *soigneurs* too. Two days without rest, preparing *bidons*, handing them up to the riders, looking after them from the back of the car which was following them. To be up to scratch some of us charged up like donkeys, mainly on Captagon.

Paris–Roubaix is the last of these crazy races. And even today many of the team managers still use the old remedies. These former bike racers know very well what they need to remain at their post behind the steering wheel. There are exceptions, of course. Someone like Bruno Roussel, for example, would never take anything, but he didn't have the same pedigree as his colleagues and in 'the hell of the North' he usually preferred to leave the steering wheel to someone else and would stand on the course somewhere to hand up a wheel or a *bidon*.

When Captagon went out of style, people moved on to Belgian mix. It's talked about a lot today, but it's been around for about fifteen years. Initially it was christened 'madman's mix' because the next day you looked as if you'd been in the nuthouse. Hardly anyone knew what it actually contained; we just knew that there were amphetamines in it. This tells you how much anyone cared, be they a rider or members of the back-up team. There were even people who injected it intravenously – just try testing the team managers as they drive along the cobbles of Paris–Roubaix – most of them will come in positive.

Later on, I even got to know a team manager, a Frenchman, who would do the injections on his riders himself. He would find out from the doctors or the *soigneurs* what the drugs would do, what time they had to be injected, and how much should be taken. Back then he couldn't afford to pay a doctor. And if you want something done properly, do it yourself.

★ ★ ★

Drugs don't only help riders to win, they can also prevent them from falling apart. In the 1983 Tour Sean Kelly was out to win the green points jersey, and one of his team mates, who was in trouble, wanted to make sure he got to the finish – both for his own self-respect and also to help Kelly. He had no choice: cortisone and amphetamines helped him to hang in there. And a lot of prayers were said to get him through the drug tests. We had the double-sided tape ready for him if necessary, but we never had to use it. He got to Paris, and Kelly kept the green jersey to the finish on the Champs Elysées.

We also came close to catastrophe during a Tour when a rider wearing the yellow jersey was in trouble. He needed some help to hang on to the lead and we decided on an injection of Synacten Delayed. As the rider said, 'On the Tour I don't mess with anything forbidden.' In his eyes, and in all our eyes, that meant detectable drugs.

The next day the rider was incapable of holding a wheel and was left behind on the smallest hill – and there were a lot of those because the stage went right through the Pyrenees. He lost the yellow jersey that day. This mistake earned me the nickname 'blocker', and those kind of nicknames stick to you for a long time. Years later on there were still people who were taking the mickey about this blunder. That year, as it happened, was a year with no big star dominant in the Tour and in such an open race the rider could have aspired to overall victory.

Paradoxically, this terrible defeat, this annihilation of all our hopes, represented a victory of sorts for those who were fighting against doping. But it was a Pyrrhic victory. With this rider it was all or nothing. And we ended up with nothing.

I often went off to take part in the round of village circuit races, the criteriums, which followed the Tour. Usually I shared a car with two of the top Belgian riders for the whole three weeks as we travelled around France. Anything went during this time, which was without rules or morals. The most explosive cocktails in the world!

The riders would often gather in bands of seven or eight, sometimes in smaller groups. They did everything together, in the same way that they decided the race result together several days before the race. After eating, this is what tended to happen: everyone who charged up would 'chip in' a little bit to a common jar. An ampoule of Pervitin, one of Tonedron, some MD. A common jar in every sense, which was mixed up before being 'served' in equal portions by subcutaneous injection. Often a snifter was kept for me so that I would be awake to drive to the next race. I remember one day, in Normandy, at the criterium in Saint Martin de Landelles, we got together in someone's house at the end of the morning. The race, if it can be called that, was to take place in the afternoon. Seated around the table were a French national champion, two Tour de France winners, two winners of the Tour of Spain, two world champions and a winner of Châteauroux–Limoges, which isn't quite in the same league.

One rider fell ill ten days before the Paris–Brussels, a race that was made for him but which, strangely, he never managed to win. He had bronchitis and treated it with ephedrine for a week – it was great stuff to clear the tubes, but had the downside that it would show up at a drug test. He stopped the course three days before the race because he didn't want to run any risks, even though the controls weren't as well run as they are now.

At the end of the race, he had to go for the drug test. There was nothing to worry about. We hid a flask of urine – kindly donated by a mechanic – in his shorts and the rider managed to dodge round the control.

A few days later, the rider had a letter from the international governing body telling him that he had tested positive on Paris–Brussels. The drug? Stimul, which was based around amphetamines. He was stupefied. I carried out some discreet enquiries and the guilty man was quickly revealed. To stay awake at the wheel of the car, the mechanic had charged up a bit, but he had forgotten. The rider was disqualified and since then that mechanic has always been careful before donating anything.

If doping was the rule, there were rare exceptions. There is one story which is completely exceptional because it's about a three-week Tour, the Vuelta a Espana, rather than a one-day race.

The rider in question turned up at the Tour of Spain with just a single year as a professional behind him and very limited ambitions. There was no leader, just a few young guys who were going to have a go on a stage somewhere. But less than a week before the finish, he took the yellow jersey. It was as unexpected a performance as it was incredible, a real feat in the face of the Spanish teams, who had never given up trying to break him. But in spite of the odds against him, he hung on. Seeing that their race was slipping away, certain teams put pressure on him to make way – dirty tricks, offers of money, threats – but the rider, who had to have two bodyguards with him for two stages, never flinched.

Well, it may seem hard to believe, but that rider never took a thing during this Tour of Spain. Nothing but stuff to help him recover. He was completely washed up by the finish, but he still won. Quite an achievement . . .

But only children remain clean, honest and devoid of second thoughts. Time teaches them about life. And that's pretty much what happened with this guy. It's hard to remain an angel in this milieu. After his resounding exploit, he occasionally gave in to the calls of the sirens. One year, when he was leader of a Spanish team, he injected a Kenacort 40 during the Tour de France. But on the other hand, he never abused it. He only accepted artificial help when he was on top form. He 'targeted'.

NINE

APPARENTLY WE LIED TO RICHARD . . .

On Friday 24 July it wasn't easy getting breakfast down. I knew that Bruno Roussel had confessed to the judge that the team had a fully organised system to provide drugs to the cyclists, and I wasn't carrying the can alone any more. Bruno's Parisian lawyer, Thibault de Montbrial, had played a clever game since the start of the scandal. He had agreed with his client that they would stay well out of the media scrum and only comment through press releases. On the Thursday, the judge had agreed to see me for three-quarters of an hour and I could tell he had believed what I'd said to him. I had already met my new lawyer, Maître Bessis, who had got a grip on all the facts in the file, and had deposited a request that I should be let out of jail. What I was worried about was how the other two people in the room – Rijckaert and Roussel – would react: would they be friends or enemies?

At eight-thirty they handcuffed me and loaded me into the van with four other prisoners. We went into the Palais de Justice by the 'mousehole' at the back of the building. I scarcely had time to catch sight of the pack of journalists baying in front of the main entranceway. Then it was down a long corridor, which opened out on a large waiting room where about twenty people were sitting. And there I saw him again for the first time since the disaster. He was sitting on a bench, his face drawn and distracted. His eyes met mine and I could read the astonishment in them. As he acknowledged me with a nod, the two policemen escorting me told me to keep moving. I hadn't seen Bruno for two weeks.

And so I ended up on the tenth floor, in a tiny room opposite Judge Keil's office. Bruno and Eric came in one after the other with handcuffs on their wrists. After years working together we sat down in oppressive silence. It finally dawned on me that during all those years we had put in we had been playing with fire.

The time I spent at RMO, from 1989 to 1992, was not spent following the rules to the letter as far as many of the riders were concerned. But back then the methods we used were very rudimentary. The riders messed about on their own, even though a new era in professionalism had begun with the Italian Francesco Moser's hour record in 1984. Covering 51.151 kilometres, he had made the previous distances seem completely risible, and had smashed the much-vaunted barrier of 50 kilometres. Moser had not raced for some time, but he had prepared with the help of Professor Conconi and the day before setting his definitive record had already smashed the old record with 50.808 kilometres. When you bear in mind that Merckx, the greatest cyclist ever, had not been able to sit down for four days after setting the previous record of 49.431 kilometres in 1972, his performance left us flabbergasted. To say the least, the Italians seemed to be well ahead of us and we had to do our best to make up the lost ground.

All the other *soigneurs* were completely baffled at how he had achieved this and we had no answer to it. All we could do was carry on in our own small way, handing out drugs to the riders who wanted them. The team doctor at RMO, Bernard Aguilanu, was completely against any artificial assistance and a proponent of clean cycling based on a healthy diet, so any organised doping programme was out of the question.

That didn't stop people leaving the clean and narrow, however. At the stage finish at Valkenburg in Holland in the 1992 Tour – a stage won by Gilles Delion, who really was Mr Clean – I came across our team leader in our plush hotel in Maastricht in deep conversation with Raymond, 'his' Belgian *soigneur* who he used when riding the winter six-day races and who was one of the old brigade, part wizard, part charlatan. Pascal Lino had been wearing the yellow jersey since Bordeaux and would keep it until the race reached Sestriere in Italy, a total of ten days. But when he caught sight of me, Pascal seemed a bit embarrassed. By the look of the plastic bag which he was trying vainly to hide behind his legs his usual preparation based on cortisone wasn't good enough for him.

After dinner, when I was making my usual round of the rooms, I found the contents of the bag spread across Lino's bed.

'So what on earth is all that lot?'

'Hey, listen, don't take it the wrong way, but he sometimes gives me the odd little thing, nothing I shouldn't use.'

Maybe not, but it was comical. Some of the ampoules were marked with a blue dot, some with a red dot, depending on 'the kind of efforts that you wanted to make'! Raymond could certainly make people believe what he wanted.

On the other hand, the arrival of Charly Mottet at RMO two years before had certainly helped to clean up the team. He was the team leader, he had more influence than anyone on the way his team mates thought and he was a rider who never wanted to know about drugs. One particular episode shows how intransigent he was on the subject. A rider invited us to his wedding reception. A special venue, big round tables beautifully set out, high-class waiter service, a four-star menu, all that jazz. Charly was sitting at the same table as me, as was an old rider. With a few glasses of wine in his guts, the old cyclist began revealing a few secrets of his days at the top. How he used to pop amphetamines by the packet, how his buttocks had so many syringe holes they looked like Swiss cheese, how he used to charge up as if he was heading for the front in Vietnam . . . Poor Charly, to start with he was embarrassed, then he just slipped out halfway through the meal.

When he arrived at RMO from the Système-U team, we knew hardly anything about him. We knew that he had the ability to win the Tour de France, but we didn't know what means we had to put at his disposal to help him get there. It was only as the races went by and we ate with him and spent time with him that we worked out what kind of a fellow we were dealing with. This was one clean cyclist. An iron supplement or an injection of an anti-oxidant (Iposotal) and that was as far as he went.

You could honestly say that Mottet was a victim of drug-taking right through his career – of other riders' drug-taking. If he had used some stuff to help him recover, perhaps only now and then, the list of races which he won – already a long one – would have been considerably longer. Who knows if he might not have won the Tour? As it was, he was a rider who was said to fall apart in the final week.

On the very few occasions that he followed a course of Medrol (an anti-inflammatory containing a small amount of corticosteroids) to clear his sinuses, he would breathe fire. He used it very occasionally for therapeutic reasons, while other guys were taking it regularly as a performance-enhancing drug. It really has to be said that Charly simply did not have the career that he merited.

It was at this time that I first met the rider with whom, over eight seasons spent together, I was to forge my closest friendship. The ties between us were stronger than between friends, more like between father and son. Ties which I thought would never break, and never change, because they were born of good nature, success and a lack of any pressure. As the races, massages and meals went by we simply became closer and closer to each other. We walked hand in hand, side by side, step in step. The rider was called Richard, and he was not the same Virenque who was to become famous in the years with Festina, still less the Virenque whom the world sees today. Life can have unpleasant twists.

It was in Japan at the world amateur road-race championship at Utsunomiya in 1990 that Richard Virenque caught the eye of Marc Braillon who had begun to promote his employment agency, RMO, through cycling back in 1986, but still knew nothing about the sport. Richard's fighting spirit may have lacked focus, but it bowled Braillon over and he forced Bernard Vallet, the then RMO team manager, to hire this hot-headed young man. Vallet was not totally convinced, but had no choice.

I remember meeting Richard for the first time in February 1991 before the Tour du Haut Var in his native south of France. We were staying at a hotel in Draguignan. Richard checked in at the wheel of a black VW Golf with two huge booming speakers on the back seat. It was like a disco on wheels. I watched him get out, with his curly hair and his John Wayne walk. I don't know why, but I liked him. He was a polite boy, a bit shy; a bit of a show-off, it had to be said, and sometimes hard to handle because he loved to get as much as he could out of life. That was how he was. He never rested. He was always talking, always messing around with this or that, his car or his cycling shoes, so much so that the other guys in the team had to lecture him about it. He was shameless about asking questions to which the answers were pure nonsense. Why should he use a 52-tooth chainring not a 53-tooth? Why use this massage cream? Why follow that racing programme? And he would listen to anyone – the mechanic, the masseur, the team manager, which just made you like him even more. Because he had such a desire to learn and go into his new profession in depth, to correct his mistakes, to get on. He reacted like a child who is learning to talk. Our working relationship just developed naturally and soon I wanted to look after him. As time went on, we became inseparable at every race we went to.

Year after year, at every level, Richard Virenque made spectacular progress. It was a shame that his tactical sense didn't develop at the same rate.

With the twenty-four-year age gap between us, we behaved more or less like father and son and he listened to me a lot, although sometimes we fell out. Even when Virenque-mania swept through France and he became a star, I never saw him like that, and he went along with me. Sometimes, during the criterium season, intoxicated with his popularity, he would ride like a fool. I would point out severely that I'd seen a few Virenques in my time. In 1996, at the Grand Prix d'Isbergues, a one-day race in northern France, he bawled me out because I didn't hand him up a bottle during the race. He didn't know that you weren't allowed to hand up bottles on the last lap of the circuit. After he'd had a tantrum in public, we talked it over in the showers. 'You've been a professional for five years but you still don't know that you can't hand up a bottle on the last lap of a race? Next time the bottle will be in your face if you're not careful.' He understood why I was outraged. Whatever happened, Richard had no side.

We respected each other for who we were, even if he knew nothing of where I'd been and of the great riders I had looked after. That wasn't his only weak area. One day, during a race, a rider was calling him the filthiest names because he wouldn't stop attacking. After the race Richard came to see me talking about a 'small dark guy from the Carrera team, number 32' whose face he didn't like. It was Claudio Chiappucci, who was ranked number one in the world around that time. And 'El Diablo' didn't hold it against Richard, appreciating that he had a lively personality and that made them rather alike.

When he lay down on the massage table Virenque would always turn back into Richard. He confided all sorts of things to me, the things that got him down, his plans, his ambitions. His dreams were all the more head-turning because he actually got to live them out. The gorgeous villa near Carqueiranne, the black Porsche, his first. Sometimes, he was more surprised than anyone at what had happened. 'Willy, sometimes I ask myself if all this is really mine.' He was spontaneous, sensitive. And I came to love Richard for all these things. And they are all reasons why his behaviour after I was arrested caused me so much pain.

How can he have forgotten his first encounter with drugs in 1993, during his first season at Festina? We were at the Criterium International, a three-stage race over two days, with a road race on the Saturday, a hilly stage on Sunday morning and a time trial on Sunday afternoon. On the Saturday Richard finished fourth, a ride which boded very well for the two stages to come. 'This evening, I want a little something,' he blurted out enthusiastically, while I rubbed his legs. 'Be careful, Richard, you've never taken anything. We don't know how your body will react to it,' I said. We had to start carefully, so it was decided that he would be injected with half a capsule of Synacten Immediate on the Sunday morning, an hour before the start. Just to see what happened. And we saw. Richard finished outside the time limit. The drug was banned from the medicine chest.

As my father always used to say, 'You don't turn a pig into a sheep by cutting his tail off.' I also remember something which Marc Madiot said in 1991, when the great rider from Mayenne was with RMO and won his second Paris–Roubaix. Richard Virenque was just a new professional, who used to poke his nose everywhere, so great was his curiosity and desire to do what the big boys did. At the training camp at Gruissan at the start of the season, in front of senior riders like Lino and Caritoux, Madiot said, 'You, my lad, will end up a *chaudière*' – cycling slang for a rider who can't stay off the drugs.

In the days of RMO, no one was really allowed to talk about drug-taking. However, as the months passed I did see some things which produced results. On one Paris–Nice, there was a good little rider who tried a cortisone injection. Up till then he had never tried anything, he was one of the clean ones. He was well up on the overall standings and asked for a Kenacort injection to put him in the best shape possible for the closing time trial up the Col d'Eze. That Sunday evening he was among the first five overall, and yet, as far as I know, this was the first and last time that he gave in to temptation.

Still on Paris–Nice: two days from the finish one year another rider finished the stage completely exhausted and was trying to work out the best way to get himself back on his feet. That evening his masseur and I decided to give him an intramuscular injection of Syncortil, a corticosteroid which, apparently, has a 'more subtle' effect than the others. Just to help him get going, you could say. The result the next day was beyond our wildest dreams: he flew like an aeroplane before winning the stage, which finished on top of a hill. We were all overjoyed, and the fact that he had to take the drug test didn't dull our delight one bit.

However, a rumour had just gained currency in the

peloton: now, it seemed, corticosteroids could be picked up by the routine urine tests. It was complete rubbish, but the *soigneur*, who was obviously concerned, sought me out in the team equipment lorry where I was getting the next day's race food ready.

'Willy, you know I gave one of the riders a bit of Syncortil today and he took the test.'

I just laughed it off. 'Don't worry, there's no problem, they can't find it.'

He wasn't convinced and thought he had been set up, so he went to warn Jacques Michaud, the team manager. He passed on the message to Bernard Aguilanu, the team doctor, who, in turn, informed Marc Braillon because he had already had his doubts about this particular *soigneur*'s way of working. The facts lost something in translation and Braillon was told that his rider had been charged up like a donkey, which was far from the truth. The *soigneur* was sacked. The rider went through the drug test without a false note and went happily on his way.

Because I worked solely with professional teams, I didn't know precisely what was going on a step or two down the ladder. A few episodes gave me a fairly exact idea, though. At the start of the 1990s during the Tour of the Vaucluse, a race open to both amateurs and professionals, I made friends with a young rider who wanted to make a name for himself during the race. He admitted that he had taken some Decca Dorabulin, an anabolic steroid which stays in the body for months and which he had injected just three days before the start. By sheer bad luck his name was drawn out of the hat for the random drug test, and he turned up like a man going to the scaffold. What happened? Nothing! He never heard anything about his sample. It is hardly likely that anyone was covering up for him, which shows that the controls are far from reliable.

In any case, the ways of the period and the interests of those involved meant there was every reason to cheat. Especially coming up to the Tour de France. In each of the teams selected for the Tour, a total of about twenty with nine riders in each, two-thirds of the line-up for the Tour would be pretty much worked out a month before the start. The few remaining places on each team would be fought over like the last seat in a lifeboat because there was usually very little to choose between any of the riders in contention. The riders up for selection would charge up during all the races in June to catch the team manager's eye to get into the Tour. During the Midi Libre, the Route du Sud, the Tour of Luxemburg, the Tour of Catalonia, the Tour of Switzerland and even the national championships a week before the Tour, the '*chaudières*' would be on full gas.

But the down side could be equally spectacular because the effect of taking drugs can be to sap the strength. Guys who had fought like demons to grab one of the last places on the Tour would see their form gradually fade during the first week of the race. This is known as the boomerang effect. On one occasion the boomerang almost caused a nasty accident as it came back. There was a French rider who was well known for his aggression on the bike and his lovely nature off it, who rarely missed out when the riders were passing round the jar. Amphetamines simply made him ten times more aggressive. One day in a stage race he got away in a group of half a dozen riders. The group took a healthy lead, but our hero simply yelled louder and louder at his companions to ride harder and harder. To make the point he began slamming his brakes on, time and again. In the car which was following them, I saw this terrifying sight: a rider who had broken away and wanted the break to go faster endangering the whole lot of them. He must have been really charged up . . .

★ ★ ★

Whether or not you were messing about, the important thing was never to get caught in the drug test. The unfortunate fate of a good French cyclist in a spring Classic bears witness to the difficulty of predicting how things would turn out. I have always felt rather responsible for this episode. Four days earlier, on the Tuesday, we had talked on the phone. The rider's motivation level was down, particularly because the lousy weather forecast for the next day meant his long training ride could well be an unpleasant affair. In a jokey tone of voice, I offered him a dose of amphetamines to make the seven-hour ride pass more quickly.

He followed my instructions and apparently had a highly enjoyable outing, but the race on the Saturday didn't go quite as he'd expected. To make matters worse he was selected at random for the drug test. In theory, there was no risk as he had taken the amphetamines some three days before and his body should have expelled them, but he still tested positive and was punished. The chances are that if he had urinated and then drunk a few pints of water before giving his sample, so that the urine that he provided was highly dilute, he would have got through the test.

The RMO chapter in my career closed with one of the finest swindles ever seen in the world of cycling. It was dirty dealing on an international level. At the end of 1992 Braillon was looking for someone to put money into the team, which he had backed for seven seasons. He thought he had come across that rare and wonderful creature, a financier willing to take the whole thing over lock stock and barrel, in the person of an Arab prince called Icham. Or that was what he said his name was.

Braillon had already taken on a psychologist, whom he called – in all seriousness – his futurologist. Our fate was in good hands. The 'futurologist' claimed to have 'a passport for the third millennium' mapped out and was working closely with the RMO employment agency. Braillon asked the man, whom he also called his 'guru', to apply his methods to the cycling team. To start with, Monsieur Guru made us change the team strip and the paint jobs on the bikes. Formerly white, green and black, they were repainted red and black. Apparently this was to scare the opposition! But we were the ones who were getting nervous. Monsieur Guru also decided that we should have a training camp in the Ardèche. No showers, no bogs and primitive living conditions. That was going too far. Led by Mottet, the riders walked out before they were made to crouch in beds of stinging nettles.

With Prince Icham, we went from marine-style boot camps to oases in the Sahara – complete with mirage. At the beginning, the arrival of this exotic personage, who had materialised out of nowhere, excited more than a few ribald comments. For his own peculiar reasons, he apparently had an ardent desire to become the patron of a professional cycling team.

The great RMO swindle took shape in Luxemburg just before the start of the Tour de France. The reputation the prince had for lavish spending was firmly established when, half an hour before dinner, the whole team was brought together in the private salon of the hotel where we were staying. Prince Icham turned up in his helicopter and met us in full regalia, turban on head, bodyguard in tow. At his side, Marc Braillon was in seventh heaven. Just think: a real prince of the blood royal. Spot on nine o'clock, we all met for cocktails provided by the prince. Marc Braillon and his team manager Jacques Michaux introduced us one by one to our potential saviour, who spoke excellent French and presented each of us with an expensive pen. It was time for the seduction to start.

It began with a short speech full of promises. The prince

would definitely buy up the whole team. There were a few curious guys who wanted to know what the sponsor would be called.

'I have so many businesses, so many options, that we haven't reached a firm decision yet.'

Prince Icham and his men turned up again later at l'Alpe d'Huez. As before, the visit was courteous and left us with grounds for optimism. To celebrate the end of the Tour he organised a massive party on a barge on the Seine with champagne flowing and dancing till dawn. We were completely at his mercy, in spite of the fact that the 'final' decision was taking some time.

The high point of this fantastic story took place the month after the Tour. Shortly before the Tour de Limousin, the whole RMO team, including all the back-up staff – about forty people in all – were invited with their families to stay in a castle near Charleroi in Belgium. Jacques Michaux explained that Prince Icham was about to announce the official takeover of the team, and it was going to be one hell of a party . . .

We were perfectly happy with the party. We were received in impressive style: a man in a suit and a pistol under his jacket asked us for our tickets at the entrance gate. Inside the grounds there were Mercedes parked all over the place. The château itself was a dream world which reeked of riches. Cocktails, caviar and foie gras were served up in a marquee and servants in livery brought in dinner. On a gold service! The meal lasted seven hours.

In his Turkish slippers and jellaba, Prince Icham went from table to table with a polite word for everyone. My wife Sylvie was sitting next to Bruno Roussel's wife and while they were talking they discovered that they were both born in 1962. Prince Icham overheard this and the *sommelier* arrived with a fine wine from 1962. The afternoon ended with singing from a Bulgarian folk group, while Prince

Icham and Marc Braillon savoured their cigars in red velvet armchairs in the front row.

But the real business still had not happened. At the start of the evening, the prince spoke to his dazzled audience, but limited himself to a new set of promises. Because some of the riders, led by Mottet, wanted firm assurances for the future, the prince, who wasn't fazed in the slightest, gave them his word that he would pay their wages. The fare had been fine, but the aftertaste was . . . well, there was something about it . . .

A few weeks later we learned from the newspapers that the famous prince was an international con man. What was kept quiet was the fact that the prince had talked Marc Braillon into giving him a large advance, which, he assured Braillon, would enable him to release from his Swiss bank account the £5 million necessary to finance the team. But Braillon cannot be blamed for being taken in – as indeed we all were – as Prince Icham was really a con man par excellence. The prince vanished into thin air, and so did a good many illusions.

TEN

X, Z, P AND THE TIME TRIAL 'SPECIAL'

On 24 July I was the first to go into the judge's office, together with Ludovic Baron. The stenographer was already waiting behind her machine. For some strange reason, I felt confident. The day before the judge had promised that I would be released at the end of the 'confrontation'.

It was at this time that I really got to know my new lawyer, Jean-Louis Bessis. He put a new dynamism into the 'confrontation', asked the right questions and brought to light the fact that the people who were really responsible were not there.

We all sat in a row in front of the judge, from left to right, Baron, me, Bessis, Bruno Roussel's lawyer Thibault de Montbrial, then Roussel himself, Dr Rijckaert's lawyer Demarcq, and finally Rijckaert. There was a prison officer at each end of the row. On the judge's left sat the procurator, a French–Flemish interpreter, Rijckaert's other lawyer and Bessis's assistant. So the stage was set and it was time for the drama to start.

This was the best, probably the only, chance to get everything out in the open – and go way beyond the Festina scandal. We only differed from other teams in two small ways: I had made the mistake of being picked up at a border post, and Roussel had made the mistake of acknowledging responsibility for his actions in public. Apart from that, we were all the same as each other. The teams are no longer made up of sportsmen, but of professionals who take all the measures necessary to do their work.

The atmosphere in the office was incredibly tense. Because we had spent more time with each other than with our families, Rijckaert, Roussel and I had become very close over the years, but the current situation had changed all that. It is not easy to defend your own interests and remain friends. The judge began by slowly reading out our statements and asking each of us for our opinions. We had to answer yes or no and expand on what had been said if necessary. I agreed entirely with Roussel's statement. What's more, during this 'confrontation', Bruno and I never found anything to disagree about. He had recognised the facts, taken responsibility and acknowledged that my place was at the bottom of the heap.

Rijckaert's version of events, on the other hand, was bound to make both of us react strongly. That morning Rijckaert stated that his role was to check the riders' health; that he had never administered any drugs to the riders; that I was the one who distributed and injected them; in other words, that he knew nothing about what had gone on. Roussel and I refuted this, but he stuck to his guns. He even claimed that he acted in an unpaid capacity in the team. I wouldn't have minded being unpaid on 6,000 francs a day. Working about a hundred days a year, it added up nicely. The judge did his sums for him. 'Not bad for a man who was unpaid,' he pointed out. Festina even paid for the doctor's end-of-year holidays, which Roussel confirmed to Judge Keil. In the middle of this argument, Rijckaert began to talk to me in Flemish. I interrupted at once, not wanting anyone to think that we were trying to confuse matters. My head was deep enough under water and I had no desire to drown.

When it was all over, the judge asked me to stay behind

with my two lawyers. I was prepared for anything. 'Monsieur Voet, I can confirm that you are free to go home at four o'clock this afternoon, but you will be placed under legal restrictions.' I could hardly believe my ears. It was as if he had told me I had won the lottery. I mumbled my thanks as I signed the release order, which he then faxed to the governor of the prison in Loos. I hardly cared about going back to my cell in the prison van, I hardly cared about the legal orders, I wasn't wearing handcuffs any more. I was free. Free in body and in spirit. Bruno Roussel had put me in the clear. What's more, he had whispered a word or two to me, 'I'm sorry Willy, but there was nothing else that I could do.' He was completely forgiven. The first reflex anyone has when catastrophe strikes is to look after themselves. I couldn't forget his sense of responsibility and his sensitivity as an employer. If a child was taking their first communion, or if someone was ill, we would automatically be given a few days off to be with our families. More than that, he seemed to respect me for the thirty years I'd spent in cycling, having been in the sport himself for only a third of that time. Bruno Roussel couldn't forget our shared history either. It was his story too.

During the winter of 1992–3 I enquired in vain about jobs with other teams; among those I approached were Jean-Luc Vandenbroucke, who ran the Lotto team in Belgium, and Bernard Quilfen, who was Cyrille Guimard's right-hand man at the Castorama team. Finally, I got a place at Festina after Pascal Lino put in a word for me, but I had to wait for more than a month. Shortly before Christmas the directors of the watch company gathered us all together, the riders and back-up staff, a total of about fifty people, in a big hotel in Andorra. We hung around in the corridor like a bunch of tarts before being led in one by one to see Miguel Rodriguez, the boss of the company, and Miguel Moreno, the team manager. Getting the riders to sign their contracts was the priority, so we kept on queuing until four o'clock in the morning. And the ones who didn't get to sign were invited back a couple of weeks later, at the start of 1993. After all the messing about we'd had with Prince Icham, our hearts were sinking, but there were no Mercedes and no sumptuous receptions to dazzle us. In the end, everything was settled on the second trip to Andorra.

The Festina team was truly cosmopolitan. It consisted of three distinct groups: the first came from RMO – Virenque, Lino, Michel Vermote, Roussel and me; the second came from the Dutch PDM team – Steven Rooks, Jean-Paul Van Poppel, Eric Van Lancker, Jans Koerts and Dr Rijckaert, who was no longer full-time; the last group was mainly Spanish and was based around the Irishman Sean Kelly. It was some tapestry. And that's why no one really hit it off. How could there be anything in common between Rooks, who was born in Friesland, and Roberto Torres, who was a child of the Madrid suburbs? Between the Dutchman Jan Gisbers, who was the team manager-in-chief, and his assistants, Miguel Moreno for the Spanish races, and Roussel for the French events? Roussel had been hired last of all mainly because the French riders led by Virenque insisted on having him, and was actually number four after Gisbers's right-hand man Piet Van der Kruis.

As their objectives were the stage races in early summer, such as the Dauphiné Libéré and Midi Libre, to build up to the Tour, the French side of the team hardly ever met the Dutch group, who were preparing for the one-day Classics at the start of the season. But at the start of June, in the Dauphiné, some of the Dutch joined up with the French nucleus to get to know them before the Tour. Steven Rooks, Jean-Paul Van Poppel and Eric Rijckaert were among these.

We came from RMO with our little batches of

corticosteroids but it wasn't long before I worked out that this was small beer compared to what was going to be set up. A few days before the start of the race, Rijckaert gave me a flavour of the 'measures' which were currently being used by certain members of the team. He needed someone he could trust to make sure that everyone followed his advice. I was the perfect candidate. Thus it was that the vague notions I had about EPO were given shape. Some of the riders had been using it since the previous year, and Rijckaert explained its effects, both bad and good. Most importantly, he told me how to use it. In actual fact, he didn't want to be involved in providing it, letting those riders who took drugs look after themselves when it came to getting hold of it. Not all riders in the Festina team took drugs but those that did were well able to look after themselves.

He also discussed EPO with Bruno Roussel, who came out against it initially. Roussel believed that riders should prepare for racing gradually, so the arrival of EPO put him in a difficult situation due to his ethical stance. But he had to give in. The question was: did we want to race to make up the numbers or did we want to compete properly, perhaps even win? Roussel could not hold out for long in the face of some team members' ambitions and the fear of being made to look a fool. The canker was in the bud.

Reality struck and buried any finer feelings at the start of the Tour, in early July at Puy du Fou in the Vendée. Before they got there, some riders knew that they could be racing on EPO. And if they did it would be a baptism of fire. Certain riders were quite fired up by the idea, particularly because the supply was free, being paid for by the team. One rider was especially pleased because he tended to get bronchitis. He had to use more EPO than the others, backed up by large injections of antibiotics to counter his viral infection.

They had no idea precisely how the EPO was going to be delivered to them. They became more and more impatient when nothing had turned up forty-eight hours before the Tour was due to start and they had to go through their pre-race medical checks. To calm down his charges, Bruno Roussel called Spain, then put down the receiver and reassured us: 'It's coming in tomorrow by plane.'

And indeed, the delivery of about a hundred doses arrived on the designated day. Dr Rijckaert became more detailed in his explanations. That day the riders concerned took a blood test in a laboratory in Cholet. Depending on each one's haematocrit level, we gave them EPO to compensate. The limit of 50 per cent had not yet been set by the UCI (it was only brought in four years later), but Rijckaert did not want to go over 54 per cent, to limit the dangers of blood clots and high blood pressure. The riders were initially permitted daily doses of 2,000 units. According to Rijckaert, this was a reasonable quantity. Then they went down to one injection every two days until about a week before the finish in Paris. There was no point in continuing the course after that because the effects of EPO are delayed.

The afternoon of the rest day in Andorra, while the team was relaxing, I was working as usual in the room which Richard Virenque and another rider were sharing. To pep them up a bit, I had set up intravenous drips of proteins, hung on hooks. The liquid was thick and had to flow very slowly into the arm, at forty drops per minute, which took a total of more than two hours.

Suddenly, the team's PR man, Joël Chabiron, burst in without knocking. This would not usually have been a problem, but he had a Spanish journalist with him. Pandemonium! We knew that although the protein drip was perfectly within the rules the journalist would just see it as doping. I flung myself at the door, put my foot in it and said that the team doctor was in the middle of examining the riders. But Chabiron didn't want to know! In a blind panic, Virenque fled into the bathroom, carrying the drip in his arm. He didn't know that it had to be kept vertical to maintain the flow of liquid. The effect of reversing the flow came at once: his blood poured back into the trip, just putting him in more of a sweat. Fortunately, while all this was going on, Joël Chabiron understood his faux pas. After closing the door I put the drip back in place and the liquid started to flow back into Richard's arm while his room mate howled with laughter.

Festina completed the Tour with a stage win (Lino at Perpignan) and fifteenth overall for another of our riders, who was the best Frenchman in the rankings. It was a result that didn't prove a great deal. We had started to use the EPO too late to achieve much more because, when a rider is racing, the haematocrit level doesn't go up easily.

A few months later, in September 1993, Pascal Hervé signed his first professional contract with the team. He was a former French amateur champion, well known for his fearless racing style, and finally had been given the chance to move to the top echelon. He didn't dither for long when it came to choosing between the little Chazal team run by Vincent Lavenu and Bruno Roussel's ambitious Festina set-up.

Once he had been introduced to the team, Hervé didn't beat about the bush when he shook my hand.

'Listen, I'm twenty-nine years old, which means I've got four or five years to earn some money with the professionals. I've said this to the doctor and I'll say it to you: don't worry about the odd injection. I know how it all works, I understand the system. There's no need to ask any questions with me.'

At the start of the 1994 season, the whole team gathered for an initial training camp at Gruissan at the end of January. It was at this time that the management and the doctors came up with an agenda, something which I had been expecting: the organisation of a system of drug provision and its financing. Bruno Roussel said, 'I have seen what's brewing in cycling. So, rather than have to shed tears if someone is unlucky and has an accident, we have decided to bring in proper medical supervision.'

The drugs concerned were EPO and a new arrival, growth hormone. It was decided that at the end of the season the cost of what each rider had consumed would be set against his bonuses and race winnings, which were shared out according to the races which he had started. The team would put up the money – about 150,000 francs. All the winnings were paid into a common account, and Joël Chabiron shared it out.

A large consumer would have about 80,000 francs set against his winnings. But, for example, in the 1997 season, which was particularly successful, we earned about 4,000,000 francs in prize money. Once the 15 per cent (about 600,000 francs) which went to the staff had been deducted, about 3,400,000 francs was left to be split between the cyclists. They didn't lose money under this system, which the press christened the 'slush fund' during the 1998 Tour.

The system was adjusted slightly a year later. We had realised that the lesser riders had trouble affording expensive drugs – an ampoule of EPO was about 450 francs, a dose of growth hormone about 550 francs – but they still contributed to the good of the team. At the request of Virenque and Hervé in particular, the riders voted by a show of hands for the equal division of the outlay on drugs. It was almost a unanimous decision. (Bassons, Halgand and Lefevre, who never took drugs, had not yet been hired by Festina.) The new professionals were there but weren't really involved and those who objected simply had to give in to the decision of the majority. The new system led to abuse, with the less talented riders using more than they needed. This meant that the gold mine was increased, and the funds went up to 600,000 francs. As a result, in 1996, Virenque and Hervé, seconded by Laurent Dufaux, wanted the team to go back to the system which had been set up two years earlier. Laurent Dufaux, who had been signed up from a Spanish team, was not in the least surprised by our system. Nor were other riders who came from opposing teams. They could not teach us anything that we didn't know already; all that varied was the system of funding. What's more, the *soigneurs* of the different teams often ended up helping each other out when we were short. There were certain colleagues on other teams with whom we would often barter a capsule of growth hormone or EPO. There was barter at a higher level as well. I've frequently sat in on discussions between the various team doctors where the same subject always came up: preparation. Essentially, everyone had the same weapons.

Even back as far as 1994, Virenque took an interest in how the EPO and growth hormone operation was proceeding. 'Do we have enough? Have you spoken about it with the doctor?' He asked so many questions, especially in the build-up to his principal aim, the Tour de France. Obviously it was in his interests that the team be as strong as possible to help him win the race, which always slipped from his fingers but which is where he became a celebrity. Virenque knew perfectly well what he was doing. His infamous 'without my knowledge of my own free will' – which is what he answered when asked if he took drugs – is a scandalous untruth.

The Festina system was kept running resolutely until 1998. The usual time, the usual place . . . All we had to do was set up the deliveries, twice a year. In February 1994 Dr Jimenez brought the first consignment to Gruissan. After that Joël Chabiron transported the doses of EPO and growth hormone from Portugal. In France, I picked them up and stored them in my vegetable basket. It would have been possible to keep them in the refrigerator at the logistics base in Meyzieu, but we felt that it was safer for me to keep them in my home. I took care of distributing them among the riders involved, depending upon their race programme and their individual needs.

Because all the riders trusted me, it was agreed that I should keep accounts of what each one consumed during the year. Hence my famous notebooks. Day by day I recorded methodically what everyone took in a year planner. I kept the planner with me wherever I went. On the diary pages I wrote the riders' names and the stuff that was given to each of them. At the end of the season I totted up their intake and passed on the end-of-year accounts to Bruno Roussel.

To prevent anyone coming across the system unawares – after all, a notebook can be lost or stolen – I used codes for the different drugs: X for a dose of EPO, underlined in red; Z, for growth hormone, underlined in blue or green. At the start of the 1998 season I had to add another P. This particular code was also used in phone conversations or any time when we might be overheard, because it stood for Clenbuterol, a cheap anabolic, which is very hard to get hold of. Joël Chabiron apparently had the necessary contacts. Virenque, Hervé, Magnien and Brochard among others had already been started on it in 1997, the year when Djamolidin Abduzhaparov, three times points winner in the Tour de France, was found positive on the Tour and was thrown off the race. Just for the record, Jean-Luc Vandenbroucke, the team manager, immediately dismissed the team *soigneur*, Laurent Van Brussel, to prove to the governing bodies that he was whiter than white. He had probably forgotten that in 1976 he was disqualified from Milan–San Remo after finishing second to Merckx because he tested positive himself.

Banned from the market in France, Clenbuterol is one of the most powerful hormones when it comes to developing muscular mass. Beef rearers are well aware of its properties: the more meat they can sell, the more money they make. It can give spectacular muscle growth. To work out its effects precisely, we needed a guinea-pig, but it couldn't be one of the riders. They are so happy to be given something new that they tend to lose all restraint and the whole *peloton* knows exactly what's happening over the next few weeks. We found the right man soon enough: me. Before the Dauphiné Libéré in 1996 I took ten pills over seven days, then urinated conscientiously into a jar from days five to eight after taking the final pill. The whole works was then sent to a laboratory in Ghent. The Clenbuterol had been eliminated from my system by day eight. For a cyclist, who will get rid of chemicals far more quickly than someone sedentary like me, the period was still shorter.

And the effects were felt almost immediately. Three hours after I took the first pill, I began shivering. I had the impression that my lungs were swelling, that I had a new battery somewhere in the system. I felt confident, full of energy, strong as a bull – on hormones. The effects lasted for more than a month, effects which we used with good results in the big Tours after that.

It was for this reason that in 1996 some French and Swiss riders did not compete in their national championships. Right then, they were in the middle of their Clenbuterol courses, and the only disastrous effects would have been those felt at the drug tests during the championships. The official reason given was a virus circulating in the team, which, according to the press, was giving us a lot of concern coming up to the Tour de France. In actual fact the whole team was at a training camp in the Pyrenees.

As a demanding endurance sport, cycling has always been a test bed for performance-enhancing substances. It didn't take me until the autumn of 1998 to find out about creatine, but this was when the newspapers went crazy about its use by footballers in Italy and rugby players in England. Creatine had been part of the cycling landscape since 1995.

Creatine is a legal substance which only builds up muscular mass if it is used in tandem with an anabolic agent such as nandrolone. It is found mainly in red meat. Without being a stimulant, it's a useful aid to endurance. Eric Rijckaert used to get it made in a laboratory in Ghent. The white powder was very costly, but you have to realise that one sachet was the equivalent of eating thirty steaks. And the day before a long time trial or a mountain stage, there were riders who would consume up to thirty grammes a day, washed down with water or yoghurt . . . Imagine sitting down to a hundred and eighty rare steaks. We had come a long way from the 1960s, when cyclists would eat a huge steak at six o'clock on the morning of a race, blissfully unaware that digesting it would devour 30 per cent of the energy they would gain from it.

As the seasons passed, many new arrivals in the team would invest in the slush fund as willingly as those who had come before them. Luc Leblanc (1994) and Laurent Brochard (1995) both came from similar milieux. When they appeared, Dr Rijckaert would always say that they had to be 'dekenakortised'. What he meant was that their intake of corticosteroids had to be drastically reduced. 'If they use corticosteroids to excess there'll be nothing left of them,' he would say. In spite of the sense of well-being which it brings, cortisone ends up destroying the muscles by increasing the demands which are made on them. This has the effect of making the tendons and joints far more fragile.

The years from 1994 to 1998 were crazy ones for the Festina team: full of success, constantly growing popularity and results which took us step by step to the head of the UCI's world team points rankings. These were the years of folly. Aside from the new boys and a few other clean riders who were left on the margins we would see the whole spectrum of drug-taking; everyone was at it, whatever team they were in. Even if some went further than others in the arms race. Remember Bjarne Riis's stunning win on the Hautacam climb in the 1996 Tour de France. The Dane, who was to win the race, literally played with his rivals before obliterating them. And the haematocrit level of his rivals, certainly at Festina, had been blithely boosted to about 54 per cent. His exploit was as perturbing for those in the know as it was spectacular to the uninitiated. Two years later from my prison cell I couldn't help laughing nervously when I saw Riis become the riders' spokesman as the Tour de France descended into farce. What kind of cycling was he defending?

To sum up, there was nothing I didn't know about what was going on in the other teams. There were other *soigneurs* who boasted about it, who thought they were big shots, convinced that they could make or break a champion. There were some who were on big bonuses from the riders whom they prepared. One of these was the Spanish masseur who had worked alongside many world-class cyclists and had offered his services to Alex Zülle at Festina. The Spaniard never made up to riders like Bassons or Medan. He had big ideas, and swore by the methods of Dr Michele Ferrari – Rominger's Italian trainer, who is now under investigation by Italian police for supplying banned substances. It was always Ferrari this and Ferrari that. I ended up having big shouting matches with him, as did Rijckaert, who was, in spite of everything we did, a believer in a certain amount of moderation.

You have to understand that by now training sessions were determined by the doses of banned drugs that riders were ingesting rather than the other way round. As soon as our backs were turned, there were Festina riders who were tiptoeing into the Spaniard's room. They just wanted to go 'faster, higher, stronger', in the words of the Olympic motto. Thus it was that Richard Virenque paid a visit to Ferrari at his home in Ferrara at the start of 1996. One consultation was enough. Richard came back in a rather perplexed state. Being prepared by the Italian would have worked out very expensive. What's more, teaming up with Ferrari was like putting a saucepan up your backside: it was immediately obvious what you were doing. And Virenque wanted at all costs to keep his family out of what he had to do. In my opinion this is the main reason why he continued to deny taking drugs even if it flew in the face of all the evidence. In the same vein, Dufaux informed me at the start of 1998 that he and this rider had consulted a Swiss doctor who had a reputation as one of the biggest 'chargers' in his profession. And they'd been going for the last two years!

But, as I always used to say over and over again: 'A champion is not made by the drugs he takes.'

Alex Zülle's arrival at the team didn't make Virenque the least bit happy. He only found out the day before the French national championship in 1997, after the news was leaked in the press. There were quite a few of us who had known about it for a week . . .

I remember that he stormed into my room that evening after dinner. 'My God, Willy, do you know what they've done? They've gone and signed Zülle.'

On the face of it, it did look as if he had been shot in the back. What was more, Zülle was to be paid a higher salary. That made sense, because he had won the Tour of Spain twice, he had been world time trial champion, and was second in the UCI's world rankings behind Jalabert. It made sense unless you were Richard. The atmosphere was stormy to say the least. The relationship between Bruno Roussel, who had been made to hire Zülle by Miguel Rodriguez, and Richard was never quite the same again. To be honest, Rodriguez had seen things as they were. For all his fighting spirit and the times he finished in the first three of the Tour (third in 1996, second in 1997), Rodriguez never saw Richard as more than an outside bet, while Zülle was a real favourite to wear yellow on the Champs Elysées in the future. Virenque was only really number one in the hearts of the crowds who flocked to the Tour. In fact, his list of wins (twelve in eight seasons if you don't include criteriums) was not quite at the level you expect from a leader paid the wages of a major star. But Richard had other things going for him: he was as impulsive as they come, he had a battling character and looked like a nice lad. Every time July came round he turned into the ideal son-in-law and the groupies' darling: in the mind of a sponsor, these assets are as important as the ability to win. No second place in the Tour de France has created as much excitement as when Richard was runner-up to Jan Ullrich in 1997. Virenque-mania reached fever pitch and Richard took to it like a fish to water.

One turning point in his relations with the fans came at the end of the 1994 Tour. Virenque had just won the first of his four King of the Mountains jerseys, and he had the worthy idea of giving all his prize money to the orphans of Rwanda. It was a gesture which turned heads throughout France. In the midst of a host of journalists who had come to bear witness to this act of generosity, which was solemnly set up in a hotel in Paris, he handed over a cheque for £25,000. A touching scene. What the press never revealed was that the idea was not Richard's – it was Miguel Rodriguez's, to increase public awareness. Virenque was just doing what he was told.

The donation was made up of all the prize money the team received during the Tour de France, and was not considered a good idea by everyone. The team's back-up staff were less than enthusiastic, as they were supposed to get 15 per cent of the winnings. With the salaries they received, the riders could afford to be philanthropists, but we were paid rather less. Seeing how unhappy we were that a large wad of cash was being whisked from under our noses, Joël Chabiron put an end to the grumbling: 'Don't worry, the big boss is paying for the whole lot.'

Three years later, the Festina team was the dominant force in the 1997 Tour de France, with Didier Rous, Laurent Brochard, on Bastille Day, and Virenque, at Courchevel, all winning stages. On every hill and every mountain pass the riders rode at the front of the bunch like a single unit. Their superiority bordered on arrogance in the final week, with the result that the German Jan Ullrich, who was an inexperienced holder of the yellow jersey, was pushed close to breaking point. This domination was not merely the result of incredible team spirit. Four months earlier the Union Cycliste Internationale had brought in the 50 per cent haematocrit limit. Since we had started using EPO, Rijckaert had insisted that the riders stay below 54 per cent, while plenty of teams were pushing their riders up to 60 per cent. So as our opponents got used to performing at the lower level, we made hay while the sun shone.

But the team missed the boat during a stage in the Vosges mountains which could have been a turning point in the Tour. At the start of the stage from Colmar to Montbeliard,

Jan Ullrich held a lead of six minutes twenty-two seconds over Virenque in the overall standings. The German had finished second to his team mate Bjarne Riis the previous year, but still had a lot to learn. Apparently taking the yellow jersey in the mountain-top finish at Arcalis the previous week had cost him a lot of strength and this showed in the final week. During a relatively innocuous climb, the Hundsruck, a threatening breakaway group formed: among them were Hervé, Rous and Virenque, but also Marco Pantani, Abraham Olano, Fernando Escartin and all the strongest riders in the race.

Ullrich was less than a minute behind, but he looked tired and the only team mate who was able to stay with him, Udo Bölts, had already worked his legs off. There was still the climb of the Ballon d'Alsace to cover, and the unthinkable looked as if it might be going to happen.

Except that, for some reason, the other riders at the front didn't want to work with us. Richard offered to pay them, but the sum he put on the table was so small that no one would move a finger, as he told me while I gave him massage that night. So instead of asking his own team mates to make the pace to gain time on Jan Ullrich, Richard – and I've never quite understood why he did this – told them to attack on their own in order for the team to win the stage. At the finish Didier Rous's stage win, with Hervé finishing second, was a glorious sight – from the outside. But it was terribly frustrating for those on the inside.

The race began to take off in earnest for Festina during the individual time-trial stage at Saint Etienne. It was on a 55-kilometre course which was sufficiently hilly to favour Virenque. He didn't think he could win it, but he at least had a good chance of limiting his losses. With this to aim for, any means were justified. The day before, Richard had heard from one of his team mates that a 'time-trial special' drug could bring him salvation. As if there is such a thing – does a 'time-trial special' have a watch in it? And does some drug company make a 'mountain special' and a 'second-category hill special'?

Richard wanted to know more. The team mate, who was one of Ferrari's protégés, told him the man to get in touch with – it was, of course, our old friend, the Spanish *soigneur*. That evening, while he was being massaged, Richard decided, after a fair bit of hesitation, that he would tell me. I tried to warn him off. With his usual treatment, EPO and growth hormone in particular, he was perfectly well prepared. Probably better than he ever had been. It only remained for us to inject a mixture of caffeine and Solucamphre at the right time to open up his lungs, which would be done the following day. In addition, because we knew nothing of what this famous 'time-trial special' contained, there was a fair chance that it would react badly with his system. However much you may want to win, if there is a chance that you can win you can't try just anything.

The Spaniard was looking after a rider from another team at that time, who had been injured, so he was available. In spite of my warnings, Richard discussed it with Bruno Roussel, who allowed himself to be persuaded. 'It's necessary for his mind,' he told me, even though he didn't sound particularly convinced. In any case, I was given the job of bringing the guy over to the hotel. The Spanish *soigneur*, who had been warned by Virenque's team mate, had already concocted the magic potion in his hotel room. He didn't mess about.

I stood there as the Spaniard launched into a lengthy sell about the various merits of the magic capsule. All I could see was a small jar without a label and a whitish liquid which could be anything and everything.

I brought the mixture back to inject it into the muscle, and carried it up to Richard's hotel room.

'There's your gear.'

'Don't be like this.'

'Listen, you can do what you like. I don't want to hear any more about it, OK?'

'Oh come on, Willy, you can make it up for me tomorrow, can't you?'

I gave in. Because I had thought of something. I was supposed to inject this rubbish into Richard's backside one hour before the start. Obviously I'd discussed it with Rijckaert, who knew nothing about what was going on, and was completely stunned. 'You can't do this,' he said. 'No one knows what the hell's in there.'

At the given moment I gave Virenque his injection. That day, he rode the time trial of his life, finishing second on the stage to Ullrich. The German started three minutes after Richard and caught him, after which the pair had a memorable ding-dong battle all the way to the finish.

'God, I felt good! That stuff's just amazing,' he bubbled. 'We must get hold of it.' Of course, his result did have something to do with the magic capsule – but there is one thing he doesn't know, unless he reads this. I had got rid of the fabulous potion and swapped it for one which contained a small amount of glucose.

There is no substitute for self-belief. The bottom line was that there was no more effective drug for Richard than the public. A few injections of 'allez Richard' going round his veins, a big hit of adoration to raise his pain threshold, a course of worship to make him feel invincible. That was the sort of gear Richard needed, and that's how it is even today.

There was, however, one story which we found hard to believe. At the end of spring 1998, a few weeks after his win in the Criterium International, Christophe Moreau was found positive. The drug? Mestolerone, an anabolic agent. It was too obvious to be true. Unlike something like nandrolone for example, which leaves no sign of its presence a week after it has been taken, everyone knows that mestolerone can be detected in the urine for at least six months. We couldn't work out what had happened.

Of course, I asked Moreau to find out more because I felt that I had done him and the team a disservice. He swore to me that he hadn't taken anything. There was just the injection that he had been given by a *soigneur* from another team the evening before the race . . . That particular *soigneur* had been up to tricks like this before. As you might expect, he put up the shutters. It was his word against Moreau's. In public Christophe stated that he had been betrayed. Without denying anything, he went so far as to compare the injection with a blood transfusion to keep him from getting AIDS. I don't bear him any grudges, he's a lovely kid. However, the craziest thing in this whole business was that three months later he was permitted to start the Tour de France because his appeal was being considered – and the governing bodies say that they are fighting doping with all their powers. In the middle of July, Moreau told the police in Lille that he had used EPO. And the sanctions for the two offences got mixed up . . .

The need to get hold of the latest drugs verged on the obsessive. From this whisper to that rumour, names of new hormones kept coming up. They might have sounded crazy, but it didn't matter what the jar contained . . . all some of the riders wanted was to become guinea-pigs for new kinds of doping. As early as 1996, IGF-1 appeared in the team. IGF, which is short for Insulin-like Growth Factor, is a growth hormone whose effects are even quicker and more spectacular. It is hard for me to say more, because I'm not a chemist, but IGF-1 soon became the in-thing.

We tried it out shortly before the world championships in 1996 in Lugano, on three guinea-pigs: Laurent Brochard,

Pascal Hervé and Laurent Dufaux. IGF-1 came in two capsules, one containing a powder, and the other a transparent liquid. The mixture gave about ten injections – either subcutaneously in the arm or stomach, or intramuscular in the buttock. It was very expensive and needed to be looked after. Between doses it had to be kept frozen and we stored it in the freezer in the team equipment truck.

Fernando Jimenez, the team's Spanish doctor, was the man who brought IGF-1 into the team, which is why it isn't in my notebooks. We used it mainly in races in Italy and Spain, particularly the Giro d'Italia and the Vuelta, where neither Rijckaert nor I tended to be with the team. It was administered in a course over six or seven days, usually in the second week of a major Tour to give a big kick to the riders' systems.

The three guinea-pigs all took to it differently. Laurent Brochard felt that it slowed him down and Laurent Dufaux didn't feel it made any great difference. Pascal Hervé, on the other hand, rode well on it. This was why we only used IGF-1 occasionally. Its benefits were far from conclusive, but it did work at least partially. Richard Virenque tried it out with Dufaux in the Tour of Romandie in 1997, but without noting any improvement. Didier Rous experimented in the Tour of the Basque Country in 1998, without any greater success. So finally we gave up on Insulin-like Growth Factor. It might have kick-started some guys, but it wasn't doing anything for the others.

There were times when doping could really be made to improve a rider's mental state, rather than the other way round, as was the case with a rider in Ghent–Wevelgem in the late 1990s. This rider is a perfectionist, with good resistance to pain, hard on himself and those around him; he's a fine professional who leaves as little as possible to chance. He was parsimonious in his use of EPO, using less than almost any rider I've ever seen. He preferred to use his head. He had worked out that he couldn't escape the system of drug provision which we had organised, but he used it above all to help his mental preparation.

He focused all his attention on Ghent–Wevelgem, which is one of the few one-day Classics apart from Paris–Tours where there is a chance of a bunch sprint finish. With this in mind he had accepted that he would have to use EPO and Soludecadron, a well-known corticosteroid regularly used in one-day races. The record books show that, on that day, he won by a whisker at the end of a suspenseful finale.

Not all the riders were as rigorous as this one. I remember that utterly lovable Swiss cyclist Bruno Boscardin. He was never ill-mannered, never said a word out of turn. A jewel. On the morning of Het Volk in 1997, like every morning, he took a Vitamin E pill to complete his build-up to the race. The trouble was that the Vitamin E was identical to another translucid yellow pill, Normison, which is a powerful sleeping tablet.

Poor Bruno gobbled down the wrong pill in the square in Ghent were the race began. He started – snoring. And 300 milligrammes of caffeine grabbed in a panic didn't make any difference. He finished the race, but nearly fell asleep on his bike.

ELEVEN

WHITE COCAINE AND A BROWN FORM

By the time I returned to Loos on 24 July, everyone in the prison had got wind of the news. In the entrance hall a warder came up to me: 'Willy, you've got to get everything ready up there. Fold the bedclothes and wash the dishes. You have to give it all in at two o'clock, but you can't leave before four.'

I still had three and a half hours to kill. They were as interminable as those which had preceded them. Serge was pleased for me. 'You're nearly out now! But you'll send us your news, won't you? It would be the first time a prisoner has written to us.' A week later he had his postcard from Veynes.

As you do when renting a property for the summer before giving up the keys, I cleaned the few square metres from top to bottom. I was stamping my feet with impatience. At a quarter to three the cell door closed behind me. I had a final look at number 237 and went down to hand my stuff in on the ground floor. 'You may take back home any personal effects which you have been given here.' No thanks! Keep the lot. I knew they would always have the smell of dirty washing no matter how clean and well ironed they were.

My two lawyers were waiting for me. I think they got on well enough, but Ludo – as I called Ludovic Baron – could feel that the affair was slipping away from him in favour of a more experienced lawyer, even though I appreciated the support he had given me. Bessis was already calling for the Tour de France to be stopped and for more people to be put under formal investigation. He was putting my level of responsibility in context and expressing his opposition to the use of drugs in sport. At four o'clock I finally smelt fresh air again. Well, not entirely. There was a vast horde of journalists, microphones and cameras blocking the horizon. We finally made it to Ludo's Renault Twingo for the trip to his home in Lille, where Sylvie and my in-laws were waiting with glasses of champagne in their hands. Ludo had organised things well. I haven't seen him since, like many other people who are only memories in the mind of someone who has cut a good many ties.

Richard Virenque was the one who suggested that I should be included in the French team for the world championship in 1994. He had already put in a word for me during the Tour de France and it was quickly settled. The French federation didn't see a problem, particularly with four riders from Festina already selected for the team – Leblanc, Virenque, Lino and Hervé. I was glad that they were prepared to put their confidence in me and I was pleased to be recognised at the highest level in a country which wasn't my own. I had only had that honour once from the Belgians, but I had worked on a day rate for the Irish team at Sallanches in 1980 and in Altenrhein in 1983.

This time I was one of five *soigneurs* recognised by the French team, which was to be the case for another four years. They were years which brought two hugely happy occasions when Leblanc and Brochard won their world titles. They were incredibly emotional times – even though I had no licence! It was not until 1997 that Charly Mottet, under orders from the national team director Patrick Cluzaud, made me take out a French licence. Cluzaud even made the point to Virenque, who answered, 'If Willy isn't with us, there's no point in selecting me.'

In every great cyclist's career, there is one definitive year. For Luc Leblanc there was no contest: it had to be 1994. First of all he won a stage in the Tour, at the top of the Hautacam climb near Lourdes, ahead of Miguel Indurain, even if 'Big Mig' didn't make life too difficult for him. And then there was his world championship win at Agrigento in Sicily, fourteen years after Bernard Hinault gave France its last world professional title. I can remember it as if it were yesterday. With Lino, Hervé and Virenque in the team, there was a nice friendly atmosphere, and all we were thinking was red, white, blue.

Since the end of the Tour, where he had finished fourth, there had been rumours that 'Lucho' was going to leave Festina. The new Le Groupement team had made him a big offer and Luc wasn't sure what to do. In fact, although he didn't dare tell anyone in the team, he was having a lot of telephone conversations with Patrick Valcke, who was the future team manager of Le Groupement, and with the PR man, Guy Mollet. Luc dithered, in a complete muddle, until the Tour of Limousin in mid-August. On the first evening of the race, while I was massaging another rider, he came into my room. 'Hey, guys, it's all sorted, I've just been talking to Bruno. Next year I'll be staying with you.' But he added in a rather distant way, 'Well, I've got to meet my agent again, but that's just a question of doing the right thing. I've made my mind up.'

He came back at about eleven p.m.

'Hey, Luc, how did it go?'

'Erm, well, I'm actually going to sign for Le Groupement.'

You can imagine the atmosphere at breakfast the following morning. Luc was a traitor; even Bruno Roussel found it hard to hide his disappointment. He didn't understand the reasons for Luc's sudden U-turn, which was not going to make things easy for him in Sicily a few days later.

When we got there the bitter feelings had not subsided. Roussel, who was staying at his own expense in another hotel, had forbidden me to look after Luc because he'd stabbed us in the back. I could understand the way my boss felt, but I was fond of 'Lucho' and I thought I'd better tell him. He threw a huge tantrum and threatened to create a scandal by telling the press. I didn't want to create ructions, so I decided to look after Leblanc without Roussel knowing. It was a sticky one.

It has to be said that the staff of the French federation really stood out in the way they refused to get involved. Every *soigneur* had to bring all the kit he needed with him to provide for the riders in his care. *Bidons*, racing caps, race food, everything . . . This went right up to the team doctor, Gérard Porte, who wanted to know how we were going to prepare the riders. The whole thing was pretty amateurish.

The rivalry between Leblanc and Virenque was born on the road and bred in the press. In that 1994 Tour Leblanc was better than Virenque, who didn't appreciate having another rider in the team become the centre of attention. The tensions between the two men were bound to get worse, even if Leblanc was about to move on. At the dinner table they tended to goad each other. There was nothing nasty in it, but it spoke volumes. And of course they ended up together in the decisive phase of the race.

At the final point at which he was allowed to take a bottle of water, two laps from the finish, Richard was pretty sure of himself. Before he grabbed the bottle from me, he put two fingers under his nose as if to say, 'I'm going to have this.' It did look as if he was stronger than Luc, even though they were both going well. Physically and mentally, Richard was at a peak. With the dose of EPO the riders had been injected with the previous Thursday, his haematocrit was at 52 per cent. And like the three other Festina riders, he had been allowed to have an intramuscular injection of 10 milligrammes of Diprostene – a corticosteroid – the day before the race, and 20 milligrammes the morning of the start. All without anyone on the Federation staff being in the know.

He was certainly strong, but Luc had fooled him and Richard admitted as much to me afterwards. As they were about to go into the last lap, he had confided to 'Lucho' that he was about to attack 'to put a minute into them'. Poor guy: within a minute it was Leblanc who went on the offensive. He was in the French team, he was a Festina team mate: Richard could not move and could only follow the chase. Half an hour later with the bronze medal around his neck, he understood that he had narrowly missed the gold, a huge victory. In a bike race, no matter how much it hurts, you must always kill off the opposition. And Richard was never able to do that.

In spite of this, the evening was one long party. Just think – a world champion and two out of three on the podium for the French team. Everyone gathered in a hotel room, the riders, the staff, the national team manager, Bernard Thevenet, and the national trainer, Patrick Cluzaud. Quite a few of those there had a shot of Belgian mix to liven them up and keep them going all night. Luc Leblanc was 'deflowered': he'd never taken amphetamines before.

I left the little gathering at four o'clock in the morning. I had to take the Australian rider Stephen Hodge to the airport and then drive home. Agrigento to Veynes in one go was about twenty hours' driving after a night without sleep. I didn't want to fall asleep at the wheel: I had an injection of amphetamines every four hours. Ah yes, my debut with the French team was indeed a memorable one.

And the world championships the next year in Colombia

were pretty memorable too. Big smiles, a warm welcome, and cocaine.

It was quite an expedition. Actually, it was a complete nightmare. Just think of the packing, the hours on the plane, the time difference. Virenque, Brochard and Hervé were among those who made the trip for Festina. We didn't take any EPO because it was going to be useless as we were spending three weeks at altitude as preparation, but we took corticosteroids, to be injected the day before the race and in the morning before the start, as in Sicily.

After having his fingers burned there, Richard was under a lot of stress in Colombia. The incredibly hilly course was made for him, but his nerves had the better of his self-belief. He decided to use some special carbon wheels, which was to cost the team its contract with its wheel supplier, Mavic. Richard borrowed the wheels which the Dutchman Danny Nelissen had used the day before to win the world amateur championship. It was not a choice which brought him luck: he was only sixth and spent the whole day chasing down breaks.

The plane home left at four o'clock in the morning, and we needed to relax while we were waiting. After dinner a large crowd of us met up in one of the team's houses for a 'grand finale' to the journey. A Colombian driver who was attached to the team had bought a block of pure cocaine for one of the staff. Four hundred francs and it was his. All that was left was to powder it with a razor blade, which just made the whole thing more exciting, and to draw out two lines, one for each nostril, on a mirror. It was like a detective novel. The cocaine was snorted through a dollar bill and those of us who had taken it were soon high. Two hours later, the euphoria faded. Our heads dropped and the remains of the cocaine were flushed down the toilet.

★ ★ ★

To understand what goes on behind the scenes, you don't have to stuff white powder up your nose. Sometimes you just have to watch the video at the right speed, for example after the world championship at San Sebastian in 1997. Ten days after Laurent Brochard won, the phone rang in my house. It was Patrick Cluzaud, the national trainer. I was out, so Sylvie gave him the number of my mobile. A little later, on the motorway in the south of France, I had a call from Charly Mottet, who was the national team manager that year.

'Hi, Willy? Come on, what the fuck is going on? What the hell were you pushing at the world's? Someone's told me that Brochard is positive.'

I almost ran into the barriers. I had looked after the three Festina riders in the team, Brochard, Virenque and Hervé, and they had had nothing which could have caused a positive test. So first of all, what was he positive for?

'They found Lidocaine in his urine.'

I knew this particular anti-inflammatory, but didn't have any in my *soigneur*'s armoury. Either it had not come from me, or there had been a mistake, but I couldn't give Charly an explanation. To get to the heart of the problem, I headed straight for the team stores at Meyzieu. As I drove, I tried to work out what could have happened. I had half an idea in my mind. Usually, Brochard was in the care of another *soigneur* in the team. I knew that he sometimes gave particular drugs to the guys he was looking after to use at races when he wasn't there. If this was the situation, Brochard took a small bag with him. The *soigneur* had been at San Sebastian off his own bat, not as part of the French team staff. This often happened at the French championship or the world championships, where there are always guys hanging around the team hotels. The national teams can point the finger at them, but can't formally stop them being there.

At Meyzieu, looking through the *soigneur*'s personal chemistry set, I came across some Inzitan, the Spanish equivalent of good old-fashioned French corticosteroids like Soludecadron. Reading the label, there was no room for doubt. The stuff definitely contained Lidocaine. And it was Lidocaine which had screwed up everything. It made you want to bang your head on the wall. I called Bruno Roussel at once, against Charly's will because he had fallen out with my team manager shortly before the world championship. The problem was that Mottet did not want to see anyone in the team hotel apart from people who were officially members of the French team. Bruno could not believe his ears. We hung up, then he called me back to tell me that we had three days to put together a medical file, that is to say to come up with a therapeutic justification for the use of the anti-inflammatory, as the UCI permits this in certain cases. I don't know who he spoke to between the two conversations.

Officially the medical certificate should have been presented when the rider took the drug test, but it seems that the UCI didn't care in the slightest if the prescription had been drawn up before or after the world championships. The important thing was to keep up appearances. And they were kept up. Laurent had been having problems with his back for a long time; he had a hernia which he hadn't wanted to have operated on and which he preferred to treat with hydrotherapy. It was a godsend. So I suggested to Bruno that we put in a predated certificate drawn up by the team's Spanish doctor, Fernando Jimenez.

This explanatory form, dated before the positive test and drawn up after it, didn't cause the international governing bodies any qualms. It was unethical — but we abandoned ethics long ago – and against their own rules. The UCI states loudly, through its president, that it is fighting doping, but it turned a blind eye to an affair which was made all the more embarrassing by the fact that it is the organiser of the world championships. In my eyes, there was only one way out left for the president responsible at the time: resignation.

On the other hand, nothing should be taken away from Brochard. Especially not his world title. When the riders set off with the same weapons from the same start line, the best man will still win. At San Sebastian, Brochard, Virenque and Hervé, the three Festina riders, all followed the same preparation: a haematocrit level a shade over 49 per cent – seven months after the 50 per cent limit had come in you couldn't really mess around – three growth hormone injections of two units each a week before the world championships; the usual corticosteroids, 10 milligrammes of Diprostene on the Friday and 20 milligrammes one hour before the start. Nothing to write home about.

But that can't be said of the evening after the victory. After a well-watered dinner at our hotel in Hendaye, just over the border, we went to a nightclub in Biarritz, where we fêted out world champion until eight o'clock in the morning. You have to be in form for a night out like that. So, before going out on the town, most of us injected a syringe full of Belgian mix. As we partied, Virenque and Hervé went around saying again and again that they wouldn't be able to race in Milan–Turin in two days' time because they would test positive. As for 'la Broche', he left us after getting involved with a friendly chap who talked him through his lousy life in a nearby bar until the early morning. There are more restful things to do before going live on the lunchtime television news. Our man in the rainbow jersey came back looking a bit out of kilter an hour before his plane for Paris took off.

TWELVE

'LEADER? NO, I'M NOT A DEALER'

A few hours after I was let out of prison, I got out of Loos, Lille and northern France. I could see sixteen days in a cell behind me in the rear-view mirror as we went down the motorway. Sylvie was driving. First of all we stopped off at her brother Patrick's house in Auxerre. There was no huge show of emotion, no real ceremony. It was just a normal meal, normal conversations, normal life. Simple, real happiness. It was all I asked.

On the Sunday morning we had to get back on the road to head for the Caritoux' house. The moment the scandal had erupted, Sylvie had been advised by the police to put the children somewhere away from it all. You never know. What's more, Sylvie had had some threatening phone calls, which were another reason to be careful. Charlotte and Mathieu could not be better looked after than with the Caritouxs at Flassan in the foothills of Mont Ventoux.

We got there early in the afternoon. Everyone was waiting impatiently, apart from Eric, because he was away on the Tour. There were tears in my eyes. Bit by bit I was putting back together my daily life, my old life, the things that mattered. I didn't want to leave it behind again. One joyful thing followed another after the tears had dried.

I don't know how to swim, but I spent the afternoon playing the fool in the swimming pool. I might fall over and get a mouthful of water, but nothing bad could happen to

117

me. I dissected the slightest movements of the people around me, the people I'd tended to gloss over before then. I had been used to spending two hundred days a year away from the ones in my life who mattered; two hundred days driving, getting on with it, without any idea how to slow down. I had to drive into a stone wall, a prison wall, to understand. I had not seen my children growing up and I was now watching them rolling around, laughing. They even helped Kim, the Caritouxs' youngest daughter, take her first steps. Who knows, perhaps this Sunday was the most magic day of my life. Thank you, Eric, thank you, Nathalie.

It was another hour and a half's drive until I reached our flat at the end of the evening. My mind was at rest and my heart was steady. I had been away for twenty-two days – exactly the duration of a Tour de France. It had been a bizarre Tour and it wasn't long before it caught up with me.

A journalist from the television station France 2 had slipped his business card under my door. He wanted to meet as soon as possible. The next morning, as I went to buy the bread, I came across an Italian reporter waiting at the entrance to the block of flats who wanted to interview me. I just wanted to get my baguette and that was all. By the time I got back from the *boulangerie*, the Italian had company. His colleague from France 2 had joined him, together with a cameraman and a sound engineer. Eventually they understood that I wanted to relax and left me in peace. Well, in peace is one way of putting it. The telephone never stopped ringing in the flat. Requests for interviews, meetings, one-to-ones, exclusives. Whenever I wanted, wherever I wanted. Suffering from battle fatigue, I put my little family in the car and we went off to stay close by at my parents-in-law, still in Veynes.

I was sitting on the sidelines when it came to the 1998

Tour de France, but I couldn't break the habit. I sat down in front of the television and watched the spectacle unfold, or rather the masquerade. The riders putting their backsides on the tarmac, pulling off their race numbers; Bjarne Riis and Jean-Marie Leblanc trying to keep together what they could. I watched Pantani dispose of Ullrich, his face like a football, on the climb of the Galibier. The German lost almost nine minutes and the yellow jersey that afternoon.

The vessel was leaking and there was no time left to bail it out. I decided to abandon ship by pressing a button. I turned the television off, disconnected the fax and telephone. They would have done better to pack up and go home as well.

By mid-August, I'd been forgotten. It was a good opportunity to go back to the cycling you know as a child, which is taken to extremes when you are an adult. My son and four of his friends had prepared a five-day stage race to the very last detail. They had thought out everything: the place and time of each stage start, the route to be followed. All I had to do was to follow them at the wheel of my car to make sure they got fed. A real course of youth hormone.

The finest stage went over the Col d'Espreaux. The Tour de France had come over here in 1986, when Jean-François Bernard won the stage finish in Gap. There were still names chalked on the tarmac. So the little narrow road over a huge blister-shaped hill became the Tourmalet or l'Alpe d'Huez. Rachid was the winner.

The last stage, on the Saturday, went down the Furmeyer, and I went in front of them so that they wouldn't take the descent at full tilt. I was a little way ahead when they all disappeared on one bend. Fati, a little Tunisian boy, had skidded on some gravel. He wasn't wearing a helmet and his long-haired skin had peeled back like a banana. The blood was pouring out of the wound and I had nothing to put on it. Fortunately, I know my first aid. While the children called for help from a nearby farm, I used my T-shirt as a compress. Fati wanted to sleep, so I just kept him talking. If his brain hadn't been made to work, he might still be there now. When the ambulance arrived, the kid's blood pressure was right down.

We had to put our holidays back. I couldn't go without knowing if the little one was beginning to get better in the hospital in Gap. After that it was too late to find a slot. Fortunately one of Sylvie's cousins offered us a fine villa with a swimming pool at Rochegude, near Bollène, while he was on holiday in Spain. It was a fair exchange: we just had to look after the house for him.

I had lost fourteen kilos since my spell in prison and my kidneys were blocked up. It was stress, the doctor told me. Those ten days were a blessing. Ten days sleeping in the sun, sipping pastis by the swimming pool, playing *pétanque* with my in-laws or football with the children. No newspapers or journalists. Apart from the occasional *l'Equipe*. You can't leave everything behind. I came home to the flat at the end of August. There were no faxes because it had been disconnected, and fortunately I don't have an answerphone. As for the post, there was nothing remarkable. Apart from a friendly letter from the local radio station, letting me know about a petition supporting me which they had got off the ground and which had been going round the area.

I didn't have any more news of Festina until September. And the news came from the bank. My salary had not been transferred into my account. I got in touch with Joël Chabiron, who assured me that he would do what had to be done. Three days later nothing had happened. I called Chabiron again and he advised me to talk to Gines Gorriz, Miguel Rodriguez's right-hand man. Gorriz explained that my pay had been cut off because I had threatened Chabiron, but there was no question of sending me a registered letter to confirm that my contract was at an end.

Clearly, Festina wanted to get rid of me without going through any legal formalities. And even today, in spite of all the legal proceedings we've gone through, I still haven't been paid for the five months which are due to me. And five months for someone like Willy Voet is about a tenth of what Richard Virenque gets in a month. So when that guy declared, as he lay by the swimming pool with his wife, that before signing with Polti he was 'the outcast of cycling' I just didn't know what to say. Nothing was strong enough.

Every year on the first Saturday in September it's the village fête in Veynes. I wouldn't have missed the bumper cars, candyfloss and the procession. At the end of the afternoon, as I was going home, a car stopped alongside. 'Are you Willy Voet? We'd like to pop in and see you tomorrow.' I don't know how to say no – that's my greatest weakness – or maybe I say it with my mouth closed so no one can hear.

Richard Virenque had accused me of being a drug–dealer back in July. Bessis had initially demanded that he retract this accusation, which was serious and libellous, but Richard and his lawyer, Gilbert Collard, did not want to know. My lawyer had warned them – if they stood by their false claim there was a risk that I 'would tell the truth about Virenque'. And that is what I did to the Swiss journalist. I explained to him that Richard took just as many drugs as any of the other Festina riders who took them. I never suspected that these words spoken over the corner of a table and published in a small Swiss magazine would unleash a media storm, which would be fuelled a few days later by a large French daily newspaper. It was 23 September, how could I forget the date? I was on my way to Paris to plead my case before a disciplinary commission set up by the

French Cycling Federation. On the way with my lawyer towards their base near the Porte de Gentilly in Paris I stopped in my tracks in front of the first newspaper kiosk I saw. My photo was the lead on the front page, next to a picture of Virenque winning at Courchevel in the 1997 Tour.

I was supposed to explain my actions when I was at Festina to the five members of the commission. I was on my own. Roussel had refused to recognise the legitimacy of the commission and the riders concerned were not summoned. As usual, Willy was left to carry the can. My lawyer insisted that the decision should be adjourned. After consulting briefly, the commission agreed to postpone its decision for two months. I had made the journey for nothing, but at least I'd seen my face on the front page.

The Willy Voet case continued to make the news. I was the only one who wanted to lift the veil and show the truth because stating the best intentions and giving lessons on morality weren't enough. Outraged by the permanent silence, I agreed to appear on television. All the to-ing and fro-ing came to a head again on 15 October, the day of my 'confrontation' with Virenque and Eric Rijckaert. 'Virenque before the judge': the final episode in the soap-opera was a big hit. Particularly when Richard was accompanied by his lawyer, the inimitable Gilbert Collard.

The two men made an entry worthy of a pair of film stars. When it came to working a crowd, they were made for each other, but when it came to the legal brief their deafening silence didn't fool anyone. At nine forty-five we all gathered in front of Judge Keil's door. Rijckaert came up in the lift reserved for detainees, his face emaciated, his cheeks livid, his wrists handcuffed. Three months in prison has you in pieces. Meanwhile, at the end of the corridor, Richard and Collard were hunched together with big smiles on their faces . . .

The surroundings were familiar, but the seating was slightly different. There were seven of us sitting opposite the judge: from left to right, Rijckaert's lawyer Demarcq, his client, Collard, Richard, Bessis, me, and Karine Mignon, Bessis's partner. Next to the judge were Portal, a colleague of my lawyer's, the interpreter and, standing next to the entry hall, a partner of Collard's. This time, I was the last to enter the room. I caught Richard's eye and he looked at me, from head to toe. Partly a bluff, but also because he was surprised. Carrying fourteen kilos less I was a different man.

I was tense as I sat down. Of course, I knew what was going to happen, but seeing Richard in a place like this, accompanied by such a lawyer, sent shivers down my spine. I was only a metre away from Richard, but we weren't Willy and Ricardo any more as in the good old days. The judge got the debate going. Virtually all the questions were aimed at Virenque. Richard stuck to his guns, or rather, his lawyer's guns: he had never taken drugs; the capsules which Rijckaert gave him only contained stuff to help him recover; he had heard rumours that there was drug-taking in the Festina team.

From where I sat, I could watch with horrified fascination as Virenque's defender played his game. Jean-Louis Bessis pointed it out to me with a nudge of the elbow. Every time the judge asked a question Collard would give Richard a bit of paper. He was simply reading out the notes. It was unbelievable. And if Collard wanted him to remain silent, he drew a line on the piece of paper. They were so well drilled. It was quite a moment of truth.

There came a point when it all got rather surreal.

The judge: 'But you must have been aware of what was going on because you were the leader in the team?'

Richard Virenque: 'Me, dealer? No, I'm not a dealer.'

Gilbert Collard: 'No, Richard, the judge said the word "leader". It's not a crime to be the team leader . . .'

123

We nearly split our sides. This was what happened when Richard was left to answer for himself. It was a telling slip. But what came next wasn't quite so funny. When Judge Keil asked Richard why his name featured in my notebook for the 1998 season, he dared to answer, 'Monsieur Voet wrote down these doses opposite my name so that he could sell them on.' As if I would use his name to cover up drug deals. Beside myself with rage, I grabbed his arm.

'You filthy liar. Aren't you ashamed of yourself? After everything I've done for you you dare to say something like that? My God, man, open your eyes. Don't you see that you're heading for the wall? Tell the truth and it will be a relief for all of us.'

Collard stepped in.

'That's enough, Monsieur Voet. You can't insult my client.'

'Getting in your way, am I?'

'I forbid you to address me using *tu*.'

'So I am getting in your way.'

I had gone too far, I admit it, and the judge had to step in to calm me down.

At the end of the confrontation, to avoid another altercation he made Richard and me leave the office separately. I waited for Rijckaert outside. When he came out we looked at each other and fell into each other's arms. Having worked out that he was heading down a dead-end street for weeks, Eric had decided to corroborate what I had said and accept his responsibility. Three days later he was released, after more than three months locked up in the prison in Douai.

That same evening Richard and Collard held a press conference . . . in the terminal at Lille Airport. In front of the press, Richard had no hesitation in saying, 'Rijckaert confirmed before the judge that he had never given any drugs to the riders of the Festina team, including me . . .'

That is exactly what Rijckaert said to Judge Keil.
Richard had forgotten the end of the sentence which the
stenographer took down, 'without their being aware of it'.

On 26 November I went back up to Paris to appear again
in front of the five-man commission which was to decide
my professional future. The press had let it be known that
the French riders who had ridden the Tour for Festina
would also be present at the Federation's headquarters in
Rosny-sous-Bois. That was why I made the journey. But I
was the only one there, with my lawyer, and we were told
that the verdict had been postponed again and I would
receive the verdict by post within ten days.

On 10 December, at about ten in the morning, Claude,
the postman, rang the doorbell. He had brought me a
registered letter from the French Cycling Federation.
Opening it, I wasn't worried, merely curious. I thought I
might end up with a six-month suspension, like the riders
who had been found to have taken drugs. Reading the first
two pages was encouraging. They were lining up with the
arguments put forward by my lawyer. I had transported
substances for doping purposes, but on the order of my
employer. I turned to the third and final page to reach the
verdict: three years' suspension.

Three years for having transported EPO and growth
hormones, banned drugs which are undetectable and thus do
not figure on the list of substances which the Union Cycliste
Internationale finds positive in drug tests. If I followed the
riders' arguments, I had not infringed the anti-doping rules
of the UCI or French Federation, which, moreover, permit
a haematocrit level of 50 per cent. Three years means for
ever at my age. Three years for talking too much, that was
for sure. I didn't understand it at all. Fortunately my judges
had showed their general, unanimous approval, or I would
have had forty years. I was deeply disgusted.

I have turned into a househusband. For someone who used to be out for more than two hundred days a year, that's quite a change. I've kept to my habit of getting up early, at about six-thirty. I get the breakfast for my wife and kids, before taking the kids to school. I come home and make the bed, do the washing-up, the dusting. Then it's out with the vacuum cleaner. Then I get the washing out of the machine and put it out to dry. I haven't learned to iron yet. About ten-thirty I pop out for a stroll with Roxane, our little dog. A quick detour to the newsagent's before my daily visit to the in-laws. A quick drink, just so I don't feel alone.

Then it's back home to get the lunch for Sylvie and the kids. I don't forget to take the pills for my high blood pressure. Then I read the paper or watch the telly. And that's it. I go round in circles, I doze, I get bored. Thank God the family is there. On my own I'd be up the creek.

EPILOGUE

April 24, 1999. The cycling season started a few months ago. A season kicking off is like spring coming again. But it's still the depths of winter for me. My lawyer fought tenaciously to have my suspension cancelled; the judge listened to his recommendations and has placed Virenque under formal investigation, together with Daniel Baal, president of the French Cycling Federation, and his vice-president, Roger Legeay, although charges against Baal and Legeay were subsequently dropped. But my lawyer's car was stolen and he has had to fight off a ridiculous case brought by Collard and his client, who claimed 100,000 francs damages and interest for having insinuated that Virenque took drugs. A few weeks ago I re-took my driving test. I'm allowed to drive again. In every other way, I'm still at the stop sign.

Through the window I watch Florent, our neighbour's son, driving his tractor. A cow gave birth early in the morning and Florent's father has a night's stubble on his face. In the quiet of my flat I can see Gilles Delion, that rider synonymous with racing 'clean' whose suitcase full of homeopathic substances used to make everyone laugh. Excuse me, Gilles, for laughing with them.

If nothing changes in the race between the drug-takers and the testers, the takers will always be a clear length ahead.

Refrigerated lorries, magic suitcases, all these little secrets have been discovered. But other ways and means have supplanted them. Unmarked cars waiting at cyclists' hotels, campervans full of fans which can travel anywhere with their fridges full of capsules hidden among the jampots, yoghurt and mozzarella. There are rumours that EPO will soon be detectable. What a result. EPO has already been overtaken by other methods of doping, based on reproducing cells and molecules. In my final weeks at Festina, Rijckaert told me about his research into the sporting applications of Interlukin (code-named IL-3), a drug used in treating certain cancers. It is a sort of growth hormone which concentrates its effects on certain muscular tissues.

It may perhaps never be proven that doping causes deaths. But the opposite will never be proven either. So I think of all the riders whose hearts just gave up: the Spaniard Vicente Lopez-Carril, dead at 37; the Belgian Marc de Meyer, dead at 32; the Belgian Geert de Walle, dead at 24; the Dutchman Bert Oosterbosch, dead at 32; the Pole Joachim Halupczok, dead at 27; Paul Haghedooren, once champion of Belgium, dead at 38; the Dutchwoman Connie Meijer, dead at 25. I think of these cyclists, whom I knew well, and I think of the others, who may have died with less fanfare as they were out training. Together with them, cycling's heart has stopped beating. How many more lives must be lost before the sport of cycling faces up to its nemesis and finally comes clean?